Monkey Business
Pain in humans and other animals

Vincent Hoogstad
Jan-Paul van Wingerden

The term 'monkey business' originated in the mid-19th century and is associated with monkeys and their mischievous and playful behaviour. Monkeys are agile, curious and like to engage in playful antics. 'Monkey business' initially referred to frivolous or deceptive activities. Over time, the meaning changed and came to describe more unethical or dishonest behaviour. For the purposes of this book, we will assume the original meaning. *Monkey Business* references the parallel origins of primates and humans, as well as the way we deal with knowledge and information. Sometimes strange antics are played with it: Monkey Business.

First press februari 2025
© Vincent Hoogstad & Jan-Paul van Wingerden
Cover illustration: Bernadette Segers-van Vlijmen
Illustrations: By the authors
Photos: See captions
Original Titel: Monkey Business
Language editing: Kirsten Anne Taylor
Published by: Freshview
Printed by: New Energy
All rights reserved. No part of this publication may be reproduced, stored in a retrieval system or published in any form or by any means without the prior written permission of the authors, nor otherwise distributed in any form of binding or cover other than that in which it was published and without a similar condition being imposed on the subsequent purchaser.

ISBN 9789083461502

'Don't let them fool ya, or even try to school ya.'

-Bob Marley

'Hey hey we're the Monkeys.'

-The Monkeys

Content

1. Preface 7
2. The Problem with Pain 11
3. Pain Stories 21
4. The Evolution of Pain 45
5. From pain to pain behaviour 59
6. How Our Pain Concept Altered 75
7. How We Deal with Pain 91
8. The Purpose of Pain 107
9. Pain as Pain Is Intended 123
10. Epilogue 153
11. Literature 161

Acknowledgements 179

Monkey Business

1. Preface

Animals like to know where they stand. In their natural, potentially threatening environment, they can relax more if what they see around them matches their expectations. In countless animal documentaries you see animals suddenly raise their heads and look around when they notice something unexpected.

Whether you like it or not, humans are animals. And humans, like animals, want to know where they stand. In their quest to have control over the world around them, humans go much further than animals. For example, humans have developed 'science'. Science is defined as 'the systematic study of the structure and behaviour of the physical and natural world through observation and experiment'. In science, assumptions or theories are tested against the evidence obtained.

There is nothing wrong with science up to this point. A problem arises when we start to apply science. Long before science even existed, people tried to understand the world around them with stories, faith and religion. Over the centuries, science has refuted or confirmed those stories. And we have come to rely on science more and more. What is sometimes forgotten is that science is not so much the 'knowing' itself but rather the process of developing and improving knowledge. Too often, things that we think we understand turn out to be different from what we thought. Science is not a smooth, paved road that we can walk with confidence. Science is a raging river with boulders of knowledge that emerge from the water here and there. Isolated chunks of information that we trust. It is not uncommon for such a boulder of knowledge to sometimes turn out to be less stable than we thought, and we unexpectedly get soaked. Science does not consist of one continuous piece of solid knowledge. Science consists of separate chunks and we are still filling the empty spaces in between with stories. These stories can give the world as it is very different, divergent directions.

That is what this book is about. About how we weave together available scientific knowledge and stories into a truth. A truth about pain. A truth that can be the real, genuine 'Truth'.

And because it is about pain, the consequences can be serious for any person with pain who receives a diagnosis, advice and treatment. A treatment with sometimes irreversible consequences. All the more reason to take a closer look at the 'truth' about pain. This book shows that it is possible to come to a different truth based on the chunks of 'hard' scientific knowledge. A truth about pain with different consequences, possibilities or choices. We do not have the illusion that what we describe in this book is the 'real' truth. We would then make the same mistake that we are questioning. That would not be smart. What we describe is another possible composition of scientific knowledge and stories, one that has a different end result.

An interesting experiment. It is up to the reader to judge to what extent we have succeeded. Enjoy reading!

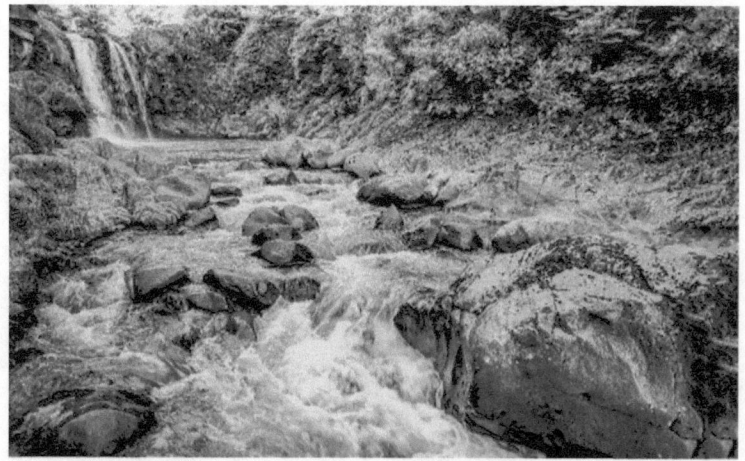

Science is like a wild river with a few knowledge rocks. The story is what we create from it. Photo: Shutterstock

2. The Problem with Pain

'We can't solve problems by using the same kind of thinking we used when we created them.'
-*Albert Einstein*

Vince: 'There's something wrong with the way we deal with pain'
JP: 'What do you mean?'
Vince: 'Well, there are so many people who suffer from pain. And despite all the research, we still don't have a cure.'
JP: 'I get that, but isn't that just the way it is?'
Vince: 'I don't think so. Because when I look at the animals that I treat, they're doing something different to what we're doing.'
JP: 'Okay, but they're animals...'
Vince: 'Aren't we?'
JP: 'You've got a point there. So you're saying that we need to look at other animals to get an idea of what we're doing wrong when it comes to dealing with pain?'
Vince: 'That's exactly what I mean.'
JP: 'Shouldn't we write this down so that others can read along with this thought experiment?'
Vince: 'That's a really good idea!'
JP: 'Well, let's get started.'

Everyday pain
We are not always aware of it, but we experience pain every day. When we get out of bed, we may feel stiff or sore. We have sore muscles from the previous day's workout, sports activity or daily work. Our gums may hurt when we brush our teeth. When drying off, we bump an elbow against the shower knob. When putting on our shoes a sore heel or toe reminds us that it takes a while to break in your new shoes.

At work we notice that our back feels stiff. At the end of the day, we are glad to finally be able to curl up on the couch and relax, tired from all the effort and discomfort we experienced during the day.

Not to mention all the little aches and pains we feel somewhere in our bodies almost every day. We don't even remember most of these little aches and pains. That's the way it should be. It's good that we forget about all these daily aches and pains. They're part of a system in our body that keeps us safe and alive. We're not supposed to feel all of these aches and pains all the time. From an evolutionary perspective, it makes much more sense to focus your attention outward, on what's going on around you. Our pain system functions as part of our safety system: it's in the background, preventing us from drinking tea that's too hot, standing on a sharp stone, bumping into objects, or pulling a muscle.

But sometimes we do become aware of our pain. This happens when the pain reaches a certain intensity, has a strange, unknown cause, or lasts longer than we expect. Becoming aware of pain introduces another aspect of that pain. In addition to simple basic protection, pain starts to shout at us: 'Hey, watch out, you're stepping into something harmful!' or 'You really should consider not doing this activity anymore!' or 'If you keep doing this, your body won't be able to keep it up for long!' These are moments when we also feel pain. And this is where the problems start. Because when we experience pain, we want to get rid of it. We can do that, as we will see later, in very different ways.

Pain affects not only the individuals who suffer daily but also our entire society. Pain is one of the leading reasons for absenteeism from work. Pain costs our society a great deal of money, not only because of the high costs incurred for medication and treatments but also because of the costs associated with absenteeism and reduced work capacity.

The number of people suffering from chronic pain continues to rise worldwide. It is estimated that 20% of adults in the Western world suffer from some form of chronic pain.

Pain is also a problem for doctors and therapists. It can be frustrating for a healthcare provider not to be able to provide relief to a patient in pain. When someone is in pain, one of our first reflexes is to want to relieve that pain. It is therefore not surprising that there are countless means and methods to reduce pain. When you enter a drugstore or supermarket, you will discover shelves full of powders, pills, ointments, sprays and potions all designed to reduce pain. Over the centuries, countless ways have been devised to relieve pain or make it bearable. These solutions range from relaxing massages, manipulations, dry needling, painkillers, opioids, electrical stimulation and TENS to denervations, fixations/fusions and even surgical removal of body parts (amputation). In addition to methods that fall within (para)medical procedures, there are also an incredible number of alternative treatment methods, ranging from homeopathic remedies to voodoo-like approaches. Some of these methods are incorporated into regular practice, including various meditation techniques known to provide some relief for patients with severe persistent pain from tumours. We do everything we can to help patients get rid of their pain. This struggle also affects the way we look at pain on a larger scale. For example, the World Health Organisation (WHO) recently officially declared chronic pain a disease in its own right and added pain to the internationally recognised list of diseases (the ICD-11 list).

Pain isn't easy
Pain is complex. Pain is not just a signal that tells us that something is wrong in our body. In addition to our physical condition, how we think and feel also contributes to how we experience our pain. Nowadays, science assumes that our nervous system can become disrupted without a clear cause and 'spontaneously' produce pain signals that we experience as pain. At least, that is what renowned pain scientists tell us. Pain therapists learn to look broadly at the histories of patients and to include

aspects from the physical, mental and social domains in their analyses.

In the past, pain was mainly seen in relation to tissue damage. Nowadays, the prevailing view is that pain mainly originates in the brain. Physiotherapists and other therapists therefore feel compelled to enter the field of psychology, in which they are often barely trained. New disciplines are evolving, which means that psychosomatic therapists are now wandering around in the obscure and vaguely defined domains between body and mind. In the field of pain management, intelligent and highly trained doctors, psychologists and therapists create complex rehabilitation programs. These programs focus primarily on behavioural and social factors. This is not necessarily a bad thing. However, physical aspects that may be related to the pain experienced are increasingly being ignored. The idea that the body could also be an avenue to reduce pain is fading into the background. If we do take a physical action, it is often severe. Pain is suppressed with medication or electricity, nerve branches are burned away, or body parts are amputated. These are extreme solutions, often with unforeseen and adverse side effects. But even simple painkillers can have serious side effects, such as stomach disorders.

How did we end up in this problematic relationship with pain? It is understandable that when we are in pain, we want this pain to go away. In our Western society, we are steadily shifting from a materialistic, physical concept of pain to a psychological approach to pain. It seems like a good idea to reconsider this one-sided path in our search for pain relief. Of course, there are social and regional differences. In the United States, the physical view is still dominant with anaesthesiologists, surgeons and the pharmaceutical industry being the main advocates.

In Europe and Australia, continued disappointment with the limited results of physical treatments in reducing pain is a major reason for an increasing call for new therapeutic approaches. The biopsychosocial lobbyists who are luring us in a psychological direction. Initially the first studies of psychological and behavioural treatments showed promising results. In the following years, however, the results of psychological treatments were found to have limitations and were less promising than initially thought.

Why is it so difficult to deal with pain? And how is it that despite all efforts and treatments, the number of people with pain is still growing rapidly?

How to deal with pain

It is strange that reducing pain is so difficult. A question we ask ourselves in this book is: are we on the right track? Perhaps we are so busy understanding scientifically and explaining the mechanisms of pain that we lose sight of its essence.

People do something with pain that we do not encounter in animals. In our Dutch pain rehabilitation clinic, the Spine & Joint Centre, people with chronic pain are treated daily. The behaviour of this patient group is largely determined by their cognitions, beliefs and emotions. Animals and humans have very similar pain systems, both biologically and neurologically. However, as Vincent experienced with animals, these cognitive-emotional factors do not seem to be that important in animals. Cats do not suffer from low self-esteem. Horses have no idea of hernias. Dogs do not feel the pressure of daily deadlines. Despite the fact that humans and animals have similar pain systems, people seem to deal with their pain very differently. What people do is not always effective, to say the least, given the huge number of people who are in pain.

> **Cognition** *is the ability to understand and acquire knowledge. This is mainly through sensory perception. Information is processed by thinking. Although the use of words and language in humans significantly enhances the cognitive process, more animals than is often assumed also have the ability of cognition.*

What are the similarities and differences between humans and animals in experiencing pain? What are the similarities and differences in how each responds to pain? Can we learn from the way animals respond to their pain?

Humans and other animals
It is time to challenge our current view of pain. We have made pain a human problem. It is not. Pain is a biological phenomenon. If we include animals in the analysis, we may get new and refreshing answers. There are countless animals that also experience forms of pain. It will benefit the discussion if we include these other perspectives on pain in our thinking. Of course, animals cannot talk. They cannot verbally express that they are in pain.
We cannot ask about their experiences.

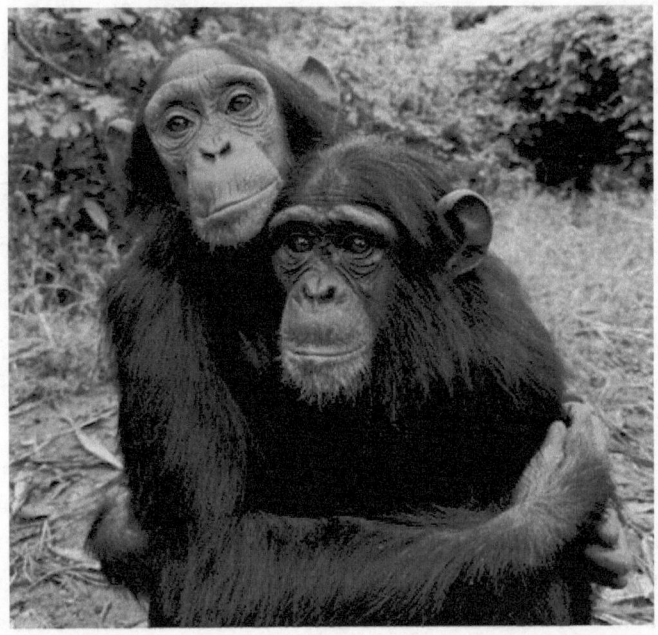

Not only people look for comfort and support. Two chimpanzees in a comfortable embrace at the Lwiro Primates Rehabilitation Center, Congo DR. Photo: Chloe Nordera

We can only observe their behaviour. By observing their behaviour, we should be able to figure out when they experience something that we would call 'pain'. There have been enormous developments in this area in recent years. As we will see, it is possible to get a sense of pain in animals. You may be surprised to learn how many animals experience pain. More interesting is the question of how they deal with or respond to their pain and what does this mean for humans? That is what this book is about. But before we dive into the technical stuff, it might be wise to first get an idea of what we mean when we talk about pain, pain perception and pain behaviour.

In the next chapter, we will start with some stories about pain. We will give a number of examples of how humans and other animals deal with their pain.

Then, we will dive into the evolution of our pain systems. By 'ours' we mean all living organisms, not just humans. It is intriguing to realise how fundamental forms of pain perception are within evolution. Without these forms of pain perception, there would be no life. The next chapter will therefore delve deeper into pain perception and pain behaviour. How do we (animals) behave when we are in pain? You will notice the complexity of pain behaviour and how strongly dependent it is on the environment.

We will also consider how our knowledge of pain has developed over the centuries. Many fundamental and exciting discoveries have been made. These findings are often accurate and correct in content. Problems arise when we translate them and want to apply them in everyday life.

With this information in our back pocket, we will look at how we deal with pain in our daily lives. Here we will see how scientific knowledge is transferred to therapeutic applications. We must warn you that this chapter contains disturbing elements. Then, we will think about the purpose of pain. The information we get from pain in animals can be very useful. With all the technical-scientific knowledge we have, we must not forget the fundamental purpose of pain.

In the last chapter, we bring everything together. We make a case for a repositioning of pain. Of course, there will always be forms of pain that need to be reduced or even suppressed. It is great to have the techniques to do that, but the main consideration is the enormous number of patients who suffer with pain from unknown causes. Perhaps as you read this book, you will discover why pain occurs. In order to reduce pain, we may have to do something completely different from what we are used to doing. There is something we can learn from our fellow animals. Will it provide a solution for every form of pain? We are afraid not. But it will certainly create new perspectives, new ideas, and yes, many human-animals will discover new ways to deal with or even reduce their pain.

3. Pain Stories

'Education is the kindling of a flame, not the filling of a vessel.'
-*Socrates*

JP: 'How are we going to do that, compare pain in humans with pain in animals?'
Vince: 'That is indeed not easy because people talk about their pain and animals do not.'
JP: 'But wouldn't it be better to look at behaviour and not at what is said? As Frans de Waal always suggested.'
Vince: 'Absolutely, we could start with some stories about pain in animals and humans, just to show what happens, like in the macaque story.'
JP: 'The Japanese macaques? I think that is a great story, Vince!'
Vince: 'Yes, it is a good example to show the impact of environment or social context on pain behaviour.'
JP: 'Pain is so much more than just an uncomfortable feeling.'
Vince: 'Yes, and these stories help to get a picture of that.'

Pain has a story

We experience pain at inopportune moments. Pain rudely interrupts what we are doing. Pain prompts us to explore a situation and tackle the problem. Most of the time, it is just a splinter, a small cut or a bruise because we bumped into something. These are the simple aches and pains that we deal with easily. There are also pains that make it more difficult for us. A headache can suddenly arise during an exciting conversation. A persistent stomach ache can occur at an inopportune moment. Or we experience back pain that constantly limits our activities. We want to do the same with this type of pain as with those other minor aches and pains: get rid of it as quickly as possible. That is easier said than done. Persistent pain never stands alone. There is always a story and only when we know the story we can understand the pain better. In this chapter, we will give some examples of pain and behaviour. Pain with a story, a history. In animals, just like in humans, pain also has a history. Behaviour also never stands alone. Behaviour changes depending on the context and the moment, but also due to knowledge, experiences and emotions.

The Story of Eva
Species: Homo sapiens; Sex: female; Age: 57; Birthplace: Rotterdam, Netherlands

As a child, Eva was already very good at gymnastics. She even competed in the national gymnastics competition. Unfortunately, she never made it to the national team. At the age of 19, she studied marketing communications, where she met her future husband, Adam. She quit her sports career, and they got married shortly afterwards. A year later, their first son Cain was born. Two years later, Abel followed. A few years later, during a holiday, Eva made a strange movement and injured her back. The pain did not go away, and Eva went to a physiotherapist. After a few sessions, her pain was gone. A few months later, the pain returned. Physiotherapy again relieved the pain, but not for long. A few weeks later, the pain returned. Concerned about this recurring pain, Eva consulted her family doctor. He reassured her that there was nothing seriously wrong and prescribed painkillers. Eva was advised to stay active and continue working. Eva continued this routine for several years, regularly seeing her family doctor, an osteopath, a manual therapist and a chiropractor, all in addition to her physiotherapy visits and always with temporary results. Eva began to worry more and more about her future.
At the age of 53, her symptoms worsen. After days of pain and being bedridden, she demands that her family doctor send her to see a specialist. The x-rays

taken by the orthopaedic surgeon show nothing other than some deformities of the lower back, which are considered normal for her age. A neurologist and rheumatologist are then consulted and find nothing. In the meantime, the pain continues to disrupt Eva's life. She goes to a pain specialist. This anaesthetist gives Eva a few injections in her lower back. After a few days of hopeful relief, the pain returns more severe than ever before. The pain specialist suggests burning off some nerve branches (denervation). Eva reluctantly undergoes this procedure. Although the doctor considers the procedure successful, it has little effect on the pain.

Eva is desperate. The GP refers her for pain rehabilitation. In this rehabilitation program, led by psychologists, Eva is expected to accept that she is in pain and to focus on what she can still do despite her pain. This evidence-based therapy is aimed at returning to work and participating in daily life despite the complaints. Eva really tries but finds it incredibly difficult to remain active when the pain does not subside. Although she is back at work, Eva is still in pain and searching for relief.

The Story of Jill and Jenny
Species: Macaca fuscata (Japanese macaque); Sex: female; Age: 3; Birthplace: Yaku Shima, Japan

Jill lives in the cold north of Japan. Jenny lives in the warmer southern region of Japan. Coincidentally, they are both pregnant and about to give birth. Jill and Jenny belong to the family of macaques, a well-known species of monkey that lives in Japan. You can recognise these monkeys by two distinguishing characteristics. Firstly, the monkeys in the cold north regularly bathe in the hot springs. There are beautiful photos of these monkeys hanging in these hot springs with the snow on their woolly heads. Secondly these monkeys are known for their habit of washing their potatoes. At first, they did this to rinse the sand off the potatoes. Later, they learned to bite holes in the potatoes and then dip them in the salty seawater. This not only cleaned the potatoes but made them taste even better. But let's go back to Jill, who is about to give birth in the north. It is deathly quiet. Jill gives birth in silence. The monkeys around her are also exceptionally quiet. The Japanese researchers who had been observing this group of monkeys for years were always surprised to see a new baby monkey. It was incredible to see how calm and quiet the births were. Initially, because of the serene course of the delivery, it was thought that these macaques had little to no pain during labour. But how different it is in the south! To the great surprise of the Japanese researchers, giving birth

in the tropical south is a completely different experience. Jenny, who lives in the south, is in labour and screams like a piglet. Many women (especially sisters and aunts) are involved in the birth. This spectacle, even if you only heard it, would lead you to conclude that Jenny is in great pain during labour.
The macaques in the north are no different physically from those in the south.

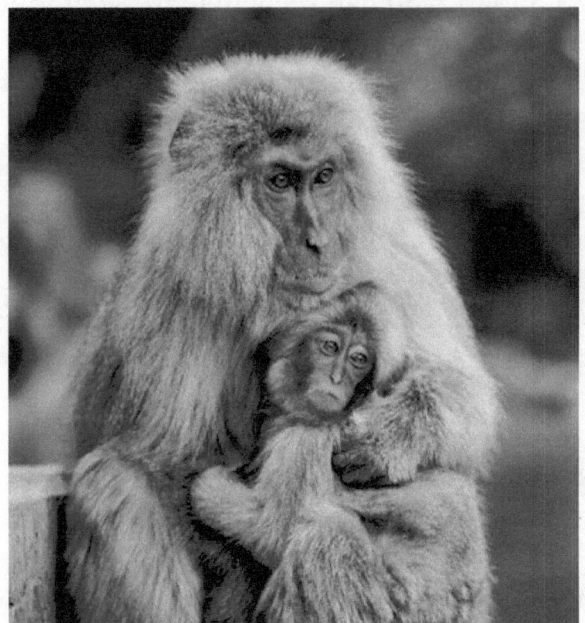

Japanese macaque (Macaca fuscata) from the colder North of Japan with kid. Photo: Shutterstock

Environmental factors and social context seem to play a very decisive role. The cold north is a harsh and rather hostile environment. The harsh climate there makes life difficult for the macaques. Food is scarce and predators are lurking. The macaques in the North are strictly led by an alpha male with a clear hierarchy. The females also function according to a strict hierarchy. This rigid hierarchy and division of roles seem to contribute to their chances of survival. Expressing pain, or rather not expressing pain, seems to increase the chance of survival here. A macaque cannot run the risk that expressing pain during childbirth or consternation in the group will attract predators.

In the South, the situation is very different. The environment is tropically warm, with always enough food. There are far fewer natural enemies. This has consequences for the structure of this group of macaques. The hierarchy is looser and more messy. There are subgroups that go their own way, and different males take the lead from time to time. This group travels widely and covers a larger area for food. Apparently, the pregnant female macaque feels no inhibition in expressing discomfort or pain, and she does so at the top of her lungs during her delivery. The other female monkeys also vocally express their excitement about the arrival of a new macaque. This also has the advantage that it is no longer necessary to send birth announcements.

The Story of Charles
Species: Homo sapiens; Sex: male; Age: 24; Birthplace: Bukavu, Democratic Republic of Congo

Charles is one of the many miners in the South Kivu region of the Democratic Republic of Congo. Working in the mines is one of the few opportunities for Charles to provide his family with a safe home and food. The work itself is anything but safe but if he finds a willing employer he will one day be able to send his children to school. Charles works hard, six days a week, and has somehow come to terms with his fate. He started working for the mine at the age of 8, cutting stones along the side of the road. Now he is an experienced miner.

On an average Tuesday afternoon, something goes wrong in the mine. A stick of dynamite unexpectedly explodes. Unfortunately, Charles is standing right next to it. He survives the accident, but his left leg cannot be saved and has to be amputated. The operation is successful, but Charles continues to suffer pain in his amputated leg. With one leg, he would still be able to work. But it is the persistent pain in his amputated leg that prevents him from working. For Charles, it is not the disability itself that limits him. Pain is his limiting factor. The pain that Charles suffers from is called phantom pain. Phantom pain is a painful sensation that a person experiences in relation to a limb or organ that is not physically part of the body, either because it has been removed or was never there in the first place. In humans, it is estimated that 60%–80% of people with an amputated limb experience phantom pain. Phantom pain is one of the forms of specific chronic pain. Although the cause is known, the amputation, it is still not entirely clear why the nervous system reacts in this way. There are therefore a number of different manifestations of phantom pain, which probably have different underlying mechanisms. Because the cause of phantom pain is not always the same, it is not easy to find a good solution. There are various forms of treatment with varying results. In a new, recent technique the nerve endings are not 'left' during an amputation but attached to a local muscle. This seems to drastically reduce the effect of phantom pain. Research into this is ongoing.

Cats and dogs are known to experience phantom pain, although we have not found any reliable and valid research on this. Due to the similar neurology between humans and animals, it seems obvious that animals can have phantom pain.

A recent study on a specific species of ant, the Florida carpenter ant (Camponotus floridanus), shows a completely different picture. Here, it is found that ants amputate the injured legs of their partners. This study is interesting for several reasons. Firstly, it shows that ants must have some form of awareness of themselves and others. In addition, biting off an injured leg of another ant requires some form of observation and even empathy: the realisation that the other is hurt and needs help. They bite off each other's (injured) legs very carefully and precisely. And they only do this in specific situations. The authors assume that they do this because these ants cannot produce their own antibiotics. Biting off the injured leg prevents infection. It only happens when the injury is close to the trunk, not when the injury is further away. Apparently, that is less dangerous. So it is a matter of survival. Unfortunately, the study does not mention whether the ants also experience phantom pain after the amputation, which would have been quite interesting in the context of this story.

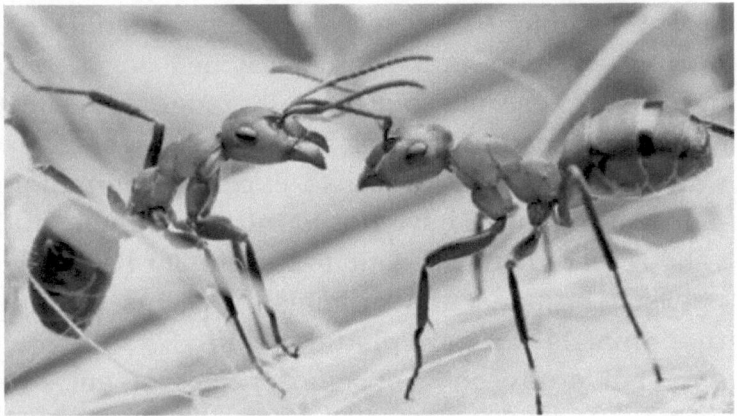

Two ants. We know from a specific ant species (Camponotus floridanus, not in the photo) that they take care of each other by biting off each other's damaged legs to prevent infection. Photo: Shutterstock

The Story of Wilma
Species: Homo sapiens; Sex: female; Age: 60;
Birthplace: Haarlem, Netherlands

Wilma, a 60-year-old athletic woman, has had a cyst on the outside of the instep of her right foot for several months. A cyst is a fluid-filled cavity that is normally harmless. This cyst did not initially cause many problems. One day, Wilma goes for a long walk. After the walk, a small infection is visible on the cyst. Over the next few days, the inflammation becomes worse. Her foot becomes red and the cyst is considerably larger. Wearing shoes is not possible.

She is advised to soak her foot in a biological detergent. This is best done in boiled water. Boiling water is, of course, much too hot, so after boiling, her partner cools the water with ice cubes to a lukewarm temperature.

During her first attempt to dip her painful foot in the water, she abruptly withdraws her foot and reproaches her partner for not having cooled the water sufficiently; it still feels boiling hot. Her partner suggests trying it with her other foot as well. Wilma can lower her healthy foot into the lukewarm water without any problem. The temperature of the water feels very different on the injured foot; the sensation is much more intense. Apparently, the inflammation has sensitised the foot considerably in just a few days. As a result, even lukewarm water is experienced as extremely hot.

Monkey Business

What is striking in this story is that the increase in sensitivity occurs within a few days. This shows that the physiological mechanism of sensitisation occurs quickly to protect a body part. Contrary to popular belief, sensitisation does not occur after weeks or months when the pain becomes 'chronic'. Sensitisation can occur immediately when this is necessary for protection.

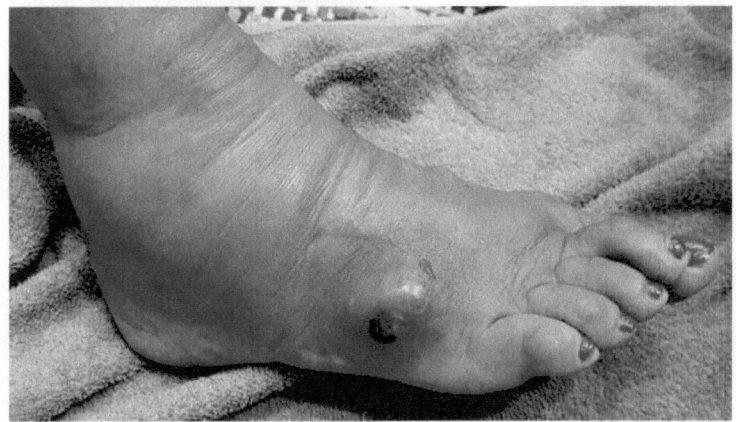

Wilma's foot (Homo sapiens, foot) was inflamed, and within a few days, the foot was so sensitised that she couldn't even bear warm water. Photo: Jan-Paul

Sensitisation: *the nervous system becoming more sensitive to stimuli.*

The Story of Chichi
Species: Pan troglodytes (chimpanzee); Sex: female; Age: 21; Birthplace: Sefadu, Sierra Leone

Chichi has been feeling unwell for a few days now. At first, she was cold and shivering. Now she feels warm, even hot. Chichi herself is unaware of it, but it is clear that she has a fever. Because she is not feeling well, she also avoids contact with her group members. She makes her way to a certain clearing in the forest. Chichi, like many of her peers, lives in a malaria-sensitive area. Chichi was probably bitten by a mosquito that carried a malaria parasite. Chimpanzees can become quite ill from malaria. In humans, symptoms include a high fever, headaches and muscle pain. Although we are not entirely sure, Chichi seems to have similar symptoms. Chichi has now arrived at the clearing. There, she shows strange behaviour. Chichi starts licking the ground. This behaviour is often seen, especially in chimpanzees suffering from malaria. An analysis of the ground that chimpanzees lick shows that this ground contains a high concentration of kaolinite. This substance is known to have a malaria-suppressing effect. Eating soil is not normal behaviour for a chimpanzee, but it is when they have malaria. They eat this kaolinite-containing soil until the malaria symptoms subside.
There is a name for eating and ingesting soil: geophagia. Geophagia occurs more often than you might think in animals and also in humans. How chimpanzees learned to eat this specific soil is

unknown. Because the behaviour is so specific and is related to having malaria, we can speak of self-medication in chimpanzees. Eating soil is a special form of self-medication. It has also been known for some time that chimpanzees, as well as other animals, actively seek out and eat certain plants that they would not otherwise eat. In the case of malaria, for example, chimpanzees eat the leaves of a certain plant, Trichilia rubescens, in addition to eating specific soil.

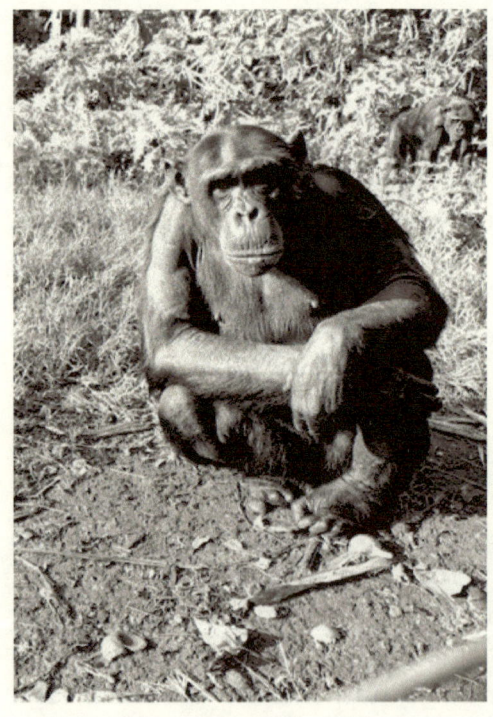

A chimpanzee (Pan troglodytes) at Lwiro Primates Rehabilitation Center, Congo DR. Chimpanzees are known to eat plants with healing properties when necessary. Many of these plants are also used in the human pharmaceutical industry.
Photo: Vincent

The Story of Sheva
Species: Ovis aries (domesticated sheep); Sex: female; Age: 4; Birthplace: Gavalochori (Crete), Greece

Sheva's delivery is not easy. The farmer has to apply extra force to her abdomen to dislodge the placenta. It should be painful, but Sheva doesn't make a sound. Even as the forceful birth pushes the intestines out, Sheva remains silent. The farmer drives the injured Sheva to the vet, completely still and alone in the back of his pick-up truck. He doesn't want to lose his precious sheep. The Cretan vet squirts half a bottle of disinfectant over the protruding intestines and then pushes them back in by hand. Without anaesthesia, Sheva's torn vagina is stitched up. All this time, Sheva is as quiet as a mouse. It's as if she doesn't mind. But that's an illusion because once back in the safety of the herd, with her lamb next to her, she bleats heartbreakingly.

To this day, it is believed that sheep feel no pain during labour. As with many other animals and even humans, this is a misconception. Sheep do experience pain, but what Sheva shows is the behaviour of a prey and herd animal. A wounded sheep is easy prey for predators. It is important that sheep do not make themselves vulnerable in threatening situations: alone, outside the herd and wounded. And expressing pain through bleating or behaviour is a sign of vulnerability. A sheep, like most prey animals, will avoid this at all costs. Until the situation is safe again. Only within the herd can what is experienced be expressed.

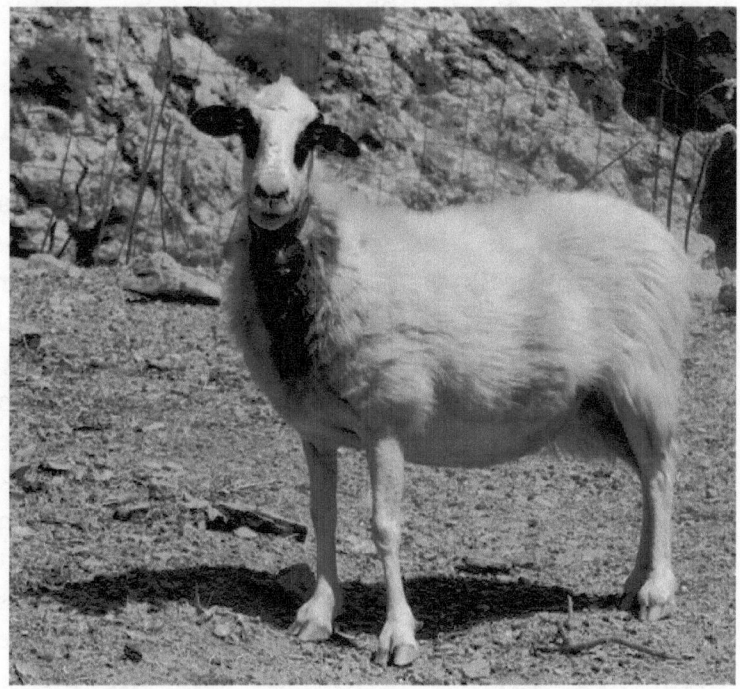

Sheep on Crete (Ovis aries). A prey and herd animal that will not quickly show its vulnerability and therefore will not quickly express when it is in pain. Photo: Jan-Paul

It is not possible for humans to estimate the pain or suffering of another human being. After all, pain is a very subjective, personal experience. This becomes even more difficult when you are dealing with animals, especially animals that are distant from us in behaviour, such as fish. If the behaviour we observe deviates from what we expect, we often do not even recognise it as pain. The neurogenic and hormonal networks of sheep are similar to those of all other mammals. It is only logical to assume that sheep experience pain in a similar way. Our pain system is no different from that of a sheep, yet there are different circumstances and behaviours. In particular, research into the psychosocial factors of pain and behaviour in sheep and other prey animals would yield interesting data.

The Story of Dory
Species: Paracanthurus hepatus – Picasso (palette surgeonfish);
Sex: female; Age: 11 Months; Birthplace: Great Barrier Reef, Australia

It was an ordinary morning at the Great Barrier Reef. Dory was swimming innocently around, waiting for a male to pass by. She had been sexually mature for a few days. Dory herself has no idea of this maturity. The only thing she feels is this vague attraction to the other side of the reef wall where a male surgeonfish is hanging out. The attraction is not unconditional. It's as if she knows the mating that is about to happen could be intense. Little by little, she approaches the other side of the reef, and suddenly, a white flash appears out of nowhere. It is a whitetip reef shark whose intention is to make Dory his breakfast. The shark's jaw snaps shut, crushing Dory as its teeth dig deep into one of her fins. In a reflex, Dory raises her dorsal fin, forcing her spines deep into the roof of the shark's mouth. The venom from Dory's spines causes a stabbing pain in the shark. The shark opens its mouth and shakes its head back and forth to get rid of the horrible feeling. Suddenly, Dory breaks free from the shark's mouth. As best she can, she swims away with her injured fin and heads for shelter. Surprisingly, Dory survives the shark's attack. But her fin remains crooked. This does not stop her from having offspring. For months after the attack, Dory avoids swimming around the area where the attack took place. And not only Dory but also her offspring are reluctant to swim around that area. The story does not say whether the shark ever chose surgeonfish for breakfast again.

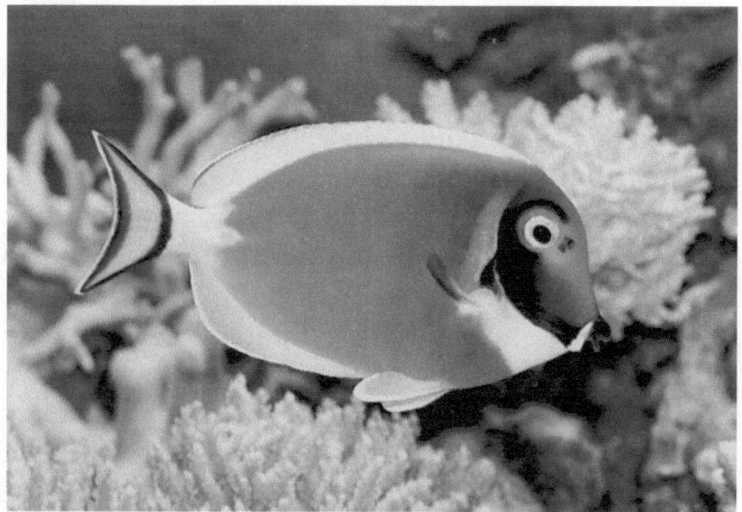

Palette surgeonfish (Paracanthurus hepatus) from the Great Barrier Reef. Fish experience sensations and pain and learn from them. The palette surgeonfish 'Dory' is one of the characters in the animated movie Finding Nemo. They have sharp and venomous spines in their dorsal fin. Photo: Shutterstock

The Story of Ellen
Species: Elephas maximus (Asian elephant); Sex: female; Age: 30; Birthplace: Periyar National Park, Kerala, India

Resigned, Ellen lowers her head and kneels. She can still remember the feeling of the training. Her skin seems thick, but it is as sensitive as that of most animals. Ellen remembers the screaming men and the stabbing pain in her side and leg, until she learned that kneeling makes the pain stop. Now, as soon as she hears the familiar cry and sees the stick next to her head, she bends her leg and kneels. To avoid that excruciating pain. Ellen has no idea that the men have hurt her on purpose to teach her to kneel and bow for the tourists. So they can take a comfortable ride on Ellen's back. Elephants may have good memories, but that is not the most important part of this story. Pain is a powerful reinforcer. And that goes for anyone who experiences pain. The experience of pain is linked to behaviour. That is why inflicting pain during animal training is an easy way to induce the desired behaviour. Pain is such a powerful coercive tool that it can result in extreme behaviour. These animals live in constant fear of the pain hanging over their heads.

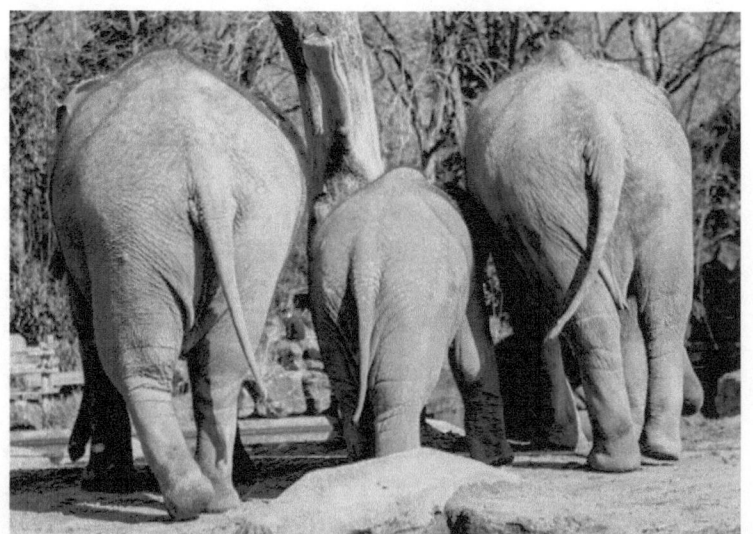
Asian elephants (Elephas maximus). Photo: Edwin Spanjersberg

The Story of Bonane
Species: Gorilla Beringei Graueri (Eastern lowland gorilla); Sex: male; Age: 30; Birthplace: Democratic Republic of Congo

It is morning in Kahuzi Biega National Park in the Democratic Republic of Congo. The dew is still on the leaves of the low forest. Bonane licks some of the refreshing dew drops from the leaves. He looks around for the others. He is now the only male among four females and three children. He recently had to chase another male, who was almost an adult, out of the group. The young silverback will have to form his own group. There is enough space in the reserve to do that, and some silverbacks roam the park alone until they find or fight for their own family.
In Kahuzi Biega National Park, people regularly come near Bonane's group. But Bonane is used to human presence. He was born into a group that was already used to the proximity of those strange pale monkeys. And because Bonane tolerates people in his environment, his descendants will do the same in the future. Because of their lifestyle, Bonane likes to look at the strange apes that pass by. Then, he can at least see what they are planning, and he doesn't have to get excited.
How different that is from the mountain gorillas (Gorilla Bereingi Bereingi) in the Virunga National Park, only 100 km further north of Bonane's habitat. Mountain gorillas live in the mountains and do not go lower than 1500 meters. As a result

their habitat is limited to the mountain on which they are born. As a result in mountain gorilla groups, several silverbacks will often live together in one group. It is necessary they tolerate each other. Among mountain gorillas, looking at each other means something different. It is not a sign of openness but a challenge. For the strange pale apes that regularly visit these groups, it is very important to know which species they are dealing with. Should they look at them or not?

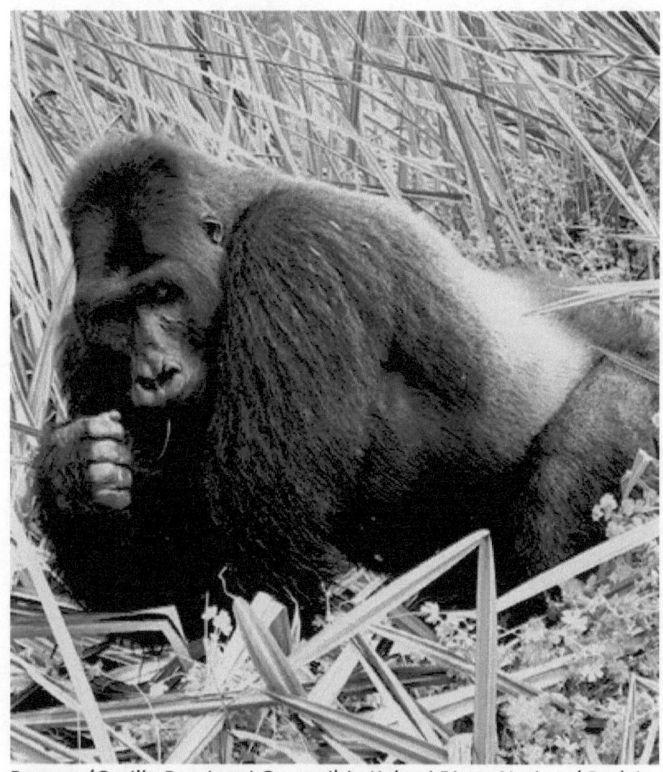

Bonane (Gorilla Bereingei Graueri) in Kahuzi Biega National Park in the Democratic Republic of Congo. Photo: Vincent

4. The Evolution of Pain

'Nothing in biology makes sense except in the light of evolution.'
-*Theodosius Dobzhansky*

Vince: 'How did it all start anyway?'
JP: 'What did all start?'
Vince: 'That humans and animals can feel something like pain.'
JP: 'Oh, that's really old.'
Vince: 'But how old?'
JP: 'Well, actually, from the very beginning.'
Vince: 'What "very beginning"? The beginning of humans or animals?'
JP: 'No, older; it started with, or maybe even before, the first single-celled organisms. Now that I think about it, shouldn't we write a chapter on the evolution of pain systems?'
Vince: 'Oh dear, are we going to go back to evolution? Do we really have to?'
JP: 'Yes, I think so. It's useful to better understand the evolutionary origin and intent of pain systems.'
Vince: 'Okay, you have a point. Let's do it then.'

Once upon a time
A creature scurries around the bottom of a warm, shallow sea. It looks like an overgrown woodlouse. We probably wouldn't recognise the animal; many of its species lived about 500 million years ago but they are no longer part of modern life on Earth. At first glance, the animal seems to wander back and forth. But if we pay close attention, we notice that it is moving steadily in a certain direction. A little further on, we see a female. Our little guy is on his way to her, irresistibly drawn in her direction because she is spreading signal hormones.

In our animal's path, a shell lies hidden in the sand of the seabed. The valves are wide open. Unsuspectingly, our animal places one of its legs in the shell, which promptly slams shut. In a reflex, the animal pulls its leg out of the shell and curls up into a ball. It is protected by its external armour plates, which completely seal it off from the outside world. For several minutes, it lies there motionless. Then, little by little, he unfolds his shell. If there is no further attack, he will continue – still timidly – on his way to the female, gracefully navigating in a large arc along the shell.

The animal in this story is fictional. It bears a slight resemblance to the abundant trilobites of a time some 500 million years ago. And although the actual trilobites are extinct, countless animals today still behave in a similar way: living, surviving and creating offspring – the basis for evolution. Living animals want to stay alive (as long as possible). They also want to reproduce. When we say 'live as long as possible', we mean living long enough to be able to reproduce and produce offspring. Some species take this very literally, such as the praying mantis, in which the female eats the male during mating.

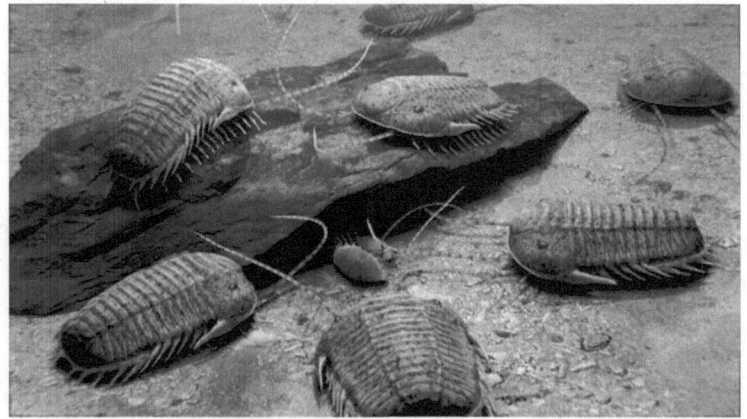

Trilobites (Trilobita) are an example of an early species able to detect (potential) damage. Photo: Shutterstock.

In our cultivated Western society, the environment is not that dangerous, but the natural world is risky and predators can lurk. A high degree of caution is required to survive. And we're not just talking about predators that want to take a bite out of us. No, we're also talking about cold, hot, salty, acidic, wet and dry conditions, all possible forms of mechanical impact that can harm our bodies. And that's not to mention all the possible insects, parasites, bacteria and viruses. Imagine getting cut, stuck, falling over something or bumping into something. In short, organisms need a system that helps them to navigate their environment without becoming too damaged. Even if you live in one place, like a plant, it is wise to keep an eye on your surroundings. For example, it is now known that even plants have mechanisms to 'know' when danger is approaching, just like insects. They can secrete chemicals to protect themselves and warn other plants in the area. Knowing what is potentially harmful around you and being able to react to it is a prerequisite for survival.

How evolution works
Let's take a moment to look at the principle of evolution. Since Darwin introduced the idea of natural selection as the basis for the theory of evolution, many have struggled with this concept. Natural selection and evolution are not a process toward perfection. It is a mistake to assume that organisms become perfect over time. Evolution has no idea of a 'perfect' that it can work towards. The process of evolution is never 'finished.' Evolution is based on the small variations that occur by chance in each individual within a species. Variations that do not increase the chance of survival will disappear. Individuals with more advantageous characteristics have a better chance of survival and produce more offspring. As a result, favourable variations will occur more often, and over time, this variation will become a characteristic of the species. Perhaps this explanation is a bit too abstract, so let's give an example. Imagine a mole in an environment with moist, soft soil. Over time, a

climate change occurs. There is less rain, and the soil becomes drier and harder. Moles with stronger front legs will be better able to continue digging through the harder ground. They can still make their holes and find food. Stronger front legs help moles survive and reproduce.

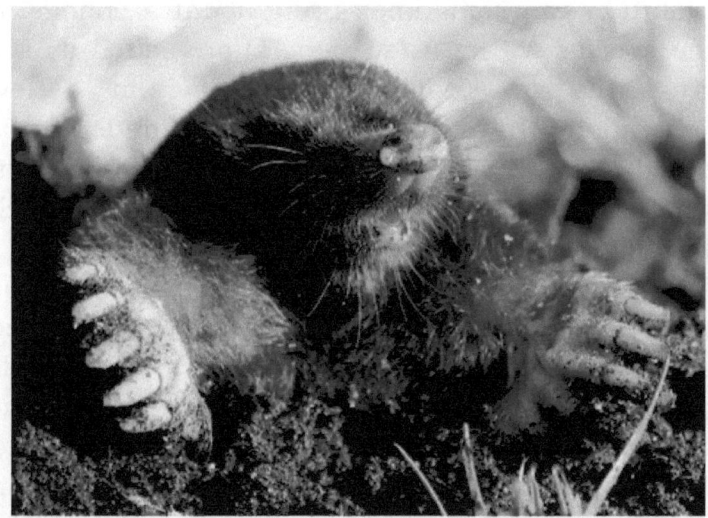

A European mole (Talpa Europaea). Environmental challenges will shape the development of a species evolutionarily, like the legs of a mole
Photo: Shutterstock

This is in contrast to the moles with weaker legs that will be less successful in producing offspring. After a few generations, the entire mole species will have stronger front legs as a characteristic. Are these stronger legs a perfect solution? No, they are not. Coincidentally, stronger legs have the advantage that the mole can continue to dig despite the drought. If the climate had become wetter instead, smaller, lighter legs with webbed feet would have been more useful.

If conditions remain more or less the same, species can remain virtually unchanged for millions of years. Take sharks, for example. Sharks are well adapted to their relatively stable environment. On the other hand, when the environment changes, evolution can sometimes bring about a change in the species within a few generations, such as the great tits in England, which, within a few generations, have started to whistle louder to be heard above the traffic noise. Male great tits that whistle louder are heard better by females, which allows for better reproduction.

This is how evolution works. It is hard to imagine that all these special, delicate and refined structures were formed by pure chance. But that is how it happens. Remember that evolution has time on its side. A lot can happen in millions of years.

Pain systems are found early in evolution. Pain systems significantly increase the chance of survival. So, pain systems are certainly not a useless remnant of evolutionary development. Pain systems are significantly important.

Nociception and pain

When we talk about the evolution of our pain system, we cannot avoid distinguishing between pain information and pain itself. What is the difference? Scientists agree that all animals have systems that can transmit pain information or nociception. These systems are necessary for survival. If you are a single-celled organism and swim in a geothermal spring because you do not perceive the damaging heat, then your survival chances decrease rapidly.

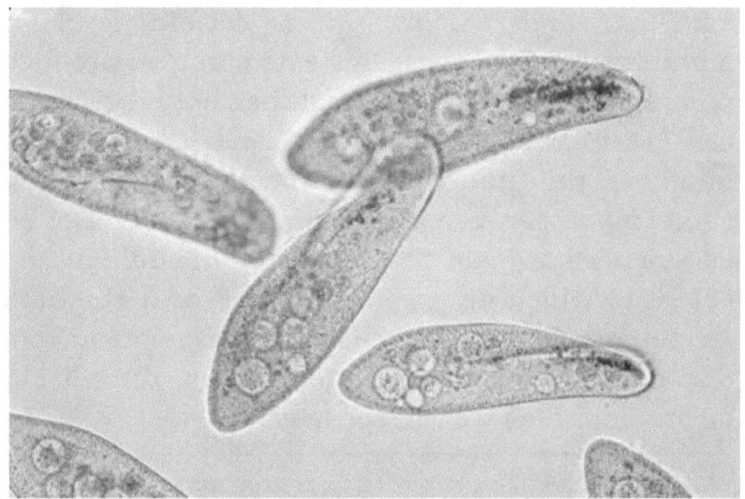

Single-celled organisms (bacteriae). Early single-celled organisms already had the ability to sense potentially harmful environments.
Photo: Shutterstock

Pain information emerged very early in evolution and is a fundamental part of all animals. It shows the essential importance of being able to perceive possible harm. By observing and recognising potentially harmful situations, an organism can adjust its behaviour and avoid the dangerous situation if necessary. To be able to recognise potentially harmful situations, sensory (nociceptive) input is needed.

Unicellular organisms can perceive simple inputs, such as temperature changes and chemical gradients. Some unicellular organisms are also sensitive to light and dark. In multicellular organisms, this input becomes increasingly specialised. Multicellular organisms can have systems for seeing, hearing, tasting, touching, smelling, and so on. At a certain level of stimulation, all of these systems can also produce pain sensations. And although perceptual systems can vary considerably from one organism to another, the underlying principle remains the same: if you can perceive something, it can also be experienced as 'pain' at some point. In addition, the extent to which an organism perceives a stimulus as potentially harmful differs between organisms and depends on, among other things, their living environment, as we will see later.

> **Nociception**: *The ability of an organism to sense tissue damage or impending tissue damage.*

From nociception to pain
The fact that an organism can perceive potentially harmful situations (nocisensory) says nothing about whether it also feels something. Pain has much more to do with experience and perception. People tend to think that experiencing pain is a very human characteristic – the general belief is that in order to experience pain, one must also have a highly developed sense of (self) consciousness. For example, it was once assumed that babies could not experience pain. After all, their self-consciousness is not yet developed. As a result, babies were

operated on without anaesthesia until well into the 20th century, whenever an operation was necessary.

Our view of the experience of pain in other animal species is also becoming increasingly understood. If a dog is bitten, it will not only try to get away, but it will also howl. This howling leads to the idea that the dog, in addition to showing a flight (or fight) response, also feels something and expresses this. That is why we believe that dogs not only have sensory skills but can also experience pain. The question then arises as to which animals can or cannot experience pain.

Within science, criteria have been established allowing us to assume that an organism experiences pain. Firstly the organism must have nociceptors. As we have seen, all animals have nociceptors, but some animals lack a central brain system. Whether having a central brain is crucial for experiencing pain is still a matter of debate. Secondly, there must be connections in the nervous system, extending from the nociceptive fibres to the higher parts of the brain. Thirdly, there must be opioid receptors, which play an important role in experiencing pain. Finally, it must be demonstrated that a) the use of narcotics suppresses a nociceptive response; b) the animal can learn from nociceptive stimuli, for example, by avoiding the situation; and c) certain normal behaviours can be postponed. All these terms are prerequisites for experiencing any form of pain. These factors have not yet been investigated in all living animals.

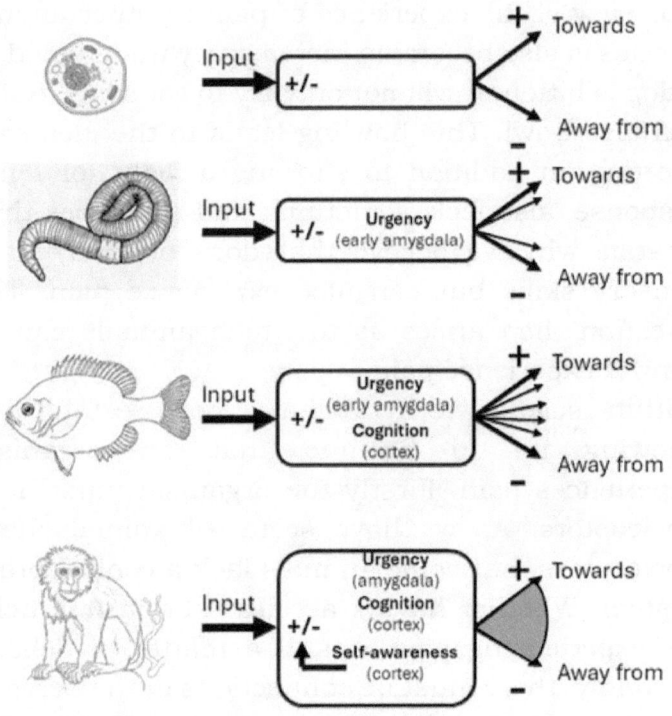

Symbolised evolutionary development of pain systems from single-celled organisms to primates. Evolutionary steps allow for a broader range of behavioural responses.

However, it is clear that these factors do apply to a great many animals, including lower animals. We can therefore conclude that all animals have a basic warning or nociception system, and many of them also have the ability to feel pain.

Nociception and behaviour

When an animal perceives a nociceptive stimulus, it will always display a certain behaviour in response. The context of the stimulus determines the nature of the behaviour, but the goal is usually to reduce or avoid the nociceptive stimulus. Nociception, in the case of physical damage, also leads to behavioural changes. For example, cuttlefish are known to keep a greater distance from predators when their legs are damaged. However, when the damaged leg is numbed, the cuttlefish swims back to the predator as if nothing had happened.

Nocisensory perception is not equally developed in all animals. For example, the naked mole rat (Heterocephalus glaber) has a limited nociceptive capacity. This animal lives in large groups underground, is cold-blooded and almost blind, and can tolerate concentrations of CO_2 that would lead to painful acidification in many animals. If the naked mole rat experienced more nociception, it would never be able to live underground.

As humans, we can experience firsthand how nociceptive perception varies greatly. Let's do a little experiment. First, pinch the skin on the inside of your forearm. Then, do the same with the relatively loose fold of skin at the tip of your elbow. You will probably notice that the elbow is much less sensitive than the forearm. The inside of your forearm has normal sensitivity. However, your elbow, like the mole rat, has a harder time because of the daily contact with hard surfaces, for example, when you work or eat at a table or desk. The sensitivity of your elbow is therefore lower than that of other parts of your body. It would be a bad idea if the nociception from your elbow were to constantly tell you that your elbow is resting on your desk.

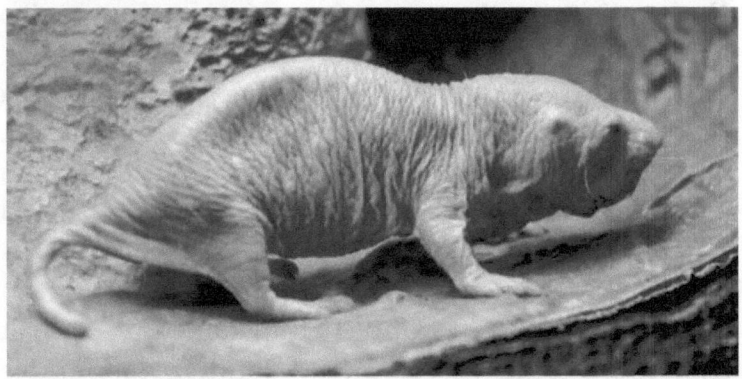

The naked mole rat (Heterocephalus glaber) has a limited nociceptive capacity, which allows it to live in very harsh environments. Photo: Shutterstock

Pain and emotion
When you ask people to name emotions, they will mention sadness, anger or frustration. Usually, these kinds of feelings also lead to certain behaviours, such as crying or approaching someone in a threatening manner. According to Nico Frijda (1927-2015), a professor of Dutch psychology, emotion is much more than just sadness or anger. Moreover, emotions are not passive experiences; they are motivators that our body calls upon to force us to take action. Emotions are more than just our 'feelings'.

There can be an internal stimulus for water or food, which can also be considered an emotional driver. However, the concepts of thirst and hunger are more often considered to be feelings: interpretations of our internal sensations.

Pain is a very powerful motivator for avoiding certain situations. The message of pain is that you have to change your behaviour to change or avoid the situation you are in – or to be very careful with it. This could well be the added value of the experience of 'pain'. If an organism has only nociception without the experience of pain, the organism will avoid the potentially harmful situation, but it will not learn from it. On subsequent occasions, the organism will behave exactly the same way until it experiences nociception. It does not learn to anticipate the potentially dangerous situation. Organisms that experience a form of pain in addition to their nociception can learn from the experience: 'I better not go that way because it makes me feel uncomfortable.' Being able to experience pain provides a much richer palette of behavioural options.

Pain perception in human and non-human animals
The basic neurological pathways for nociception are very old. As far as we could find, all animals have some form of nociception. Experiencing nocisensory information does not lead to pain in all animal species – as far as can be scientifically determined. However, the number of animal species that do

experience pain is greater than generally assumed. Although some scientists use a stricter definition, we could say that all animals with a central nervous system and the ability to learn and adapt their behaviour can experience some form of pain. This also means that the basis of the human pain system is very similar to that of other animal species. Just like us, all these animals have the ability to experience pain.

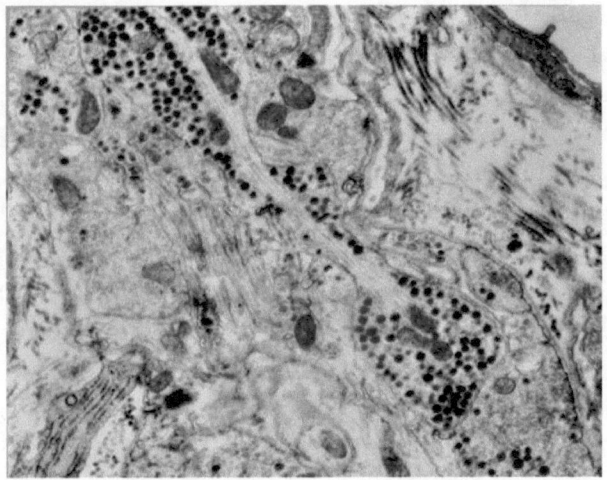

Electron micrograph of the base of the hypothalamus of a rat with dozens of nerve cell extensions. The black vesicles contain hormones (oxytocin or vasopressin). Microscopically, there is ample difference between the nervous system of humans and rats. Photo: Rob Stoeckart, PhD, Erasmus University

If the differences between us and other species with regard to pain systems are so small, why do we humans react so differently to pain than other animals? Could it have something to do with the way we talk about pain? We will investigate this further in the next chapter.

5. From pain to pain behaviour

'Those who proclaim that "animals are not people" tend to forget that, while this is true, it is equally true that people are animals. Minimizing the complexity of animal behaviour without doing the same for human behaviour creates an artificial barrier.'
-*Frans de Waal*

Vince: 'Social interactions and culture have a strong influence on pain behaviour.'
JP: 'Huh, I thought pain was a personal, emotional experience.'
Vince: 'That's true, but our social interactions and the culture we live in largely determine how we respond to pain and how we experience or express it.'
JP: 'Okay, are you talking about humans?'
Vince: 'Yes, you would think so, but you'd be surprised how much this also applies to animals.'
JP: 'Can you tell me more about how culture influences pain behaviour? And how it applies to both human and non-human animals.'
Vince: 'I have a better idea; let's dedicate a chapter to it!'

Behaviour and Culture
In Chapter 3, you read the story of Jill and Jenny, the two young macaque mothers. Both live in Japan – one in the cold north, the other in the warm south. Using this story, we illustrated how the environment influences (pain) behaviour.
In behavioural biology, it is assumed that behaviour always has a reason. In early evolutionary thinking, it was assumed that survival (eating and reproducing) was the most important driving force behind behaviour. But the more the behaviour of animals is studied, the more it becomes clear that there can be very different motivators for behaviour. This is especially evident in the more social animal species. Other important motivators are, for example, determining social hierarchy, safety, comfortable living and sleeping. Playing, learning and having fun also play a part in this and therefore are important drivers for behaviour. What we call 'just having fun' is important for development and social relationships and a good reason for certain behaviour. This applies equally to human animals.
As mentioned, the environment is an important determining factor for behaviour. This environment includes members of the same species, other species, climate, availability of food types, seasons, and so on. A hostile, dangerous environment will lead to different behaviour than a safe environment with sufficient food and protection. When circumstances change, behaviour can also change. Within a stable environment, Behaviour will not

change quickly. Stable behaviour can become a habit, even become embedded in the culture.

What is 'culture' anyway? According to the dictionary definition, culture is the set of norms, values, traditions, rules and artistic expressions of a country, people or group. In addition, culture can also mean 'art', the cultivation of crops or bacteria that are grown on a nutrient medium. Within the context of this book, we use the first definition. This definition of culture is defined with humans implicitly in mind. Could there be such a thing as culture in animals? Yes, absolutely. The definition of culture in animals is defined as the available information that can influence the behaviour of individuals. This information is transmitted by conspecifics through imitation or other forms of social transmission. Think of macaques, who learn from generation to generation to take warm baths to protect themselves from the cold. They not only wash potatoes, but they also bite into them, allowing salty seawater to penetrate deeper into the potato. Dolphins (Tursiops aduncus, Shark Bay, Australia) have been sticking sea sponges on their snouts for protection for generations. With these sea sponges on their noses, stones or poisonous coral do not rub up against their snouts when they dig up the seabed. Generation after generation passes on information about things like hunting techniques, migration routes, suitable fishing spots, preparing food or seduction tricks. Even caring for offspring appears to be a learned skill. We have been talking about behaviour for a while now.

But what exactly do we mean by behaviour? And is behaviour something that also evolves?

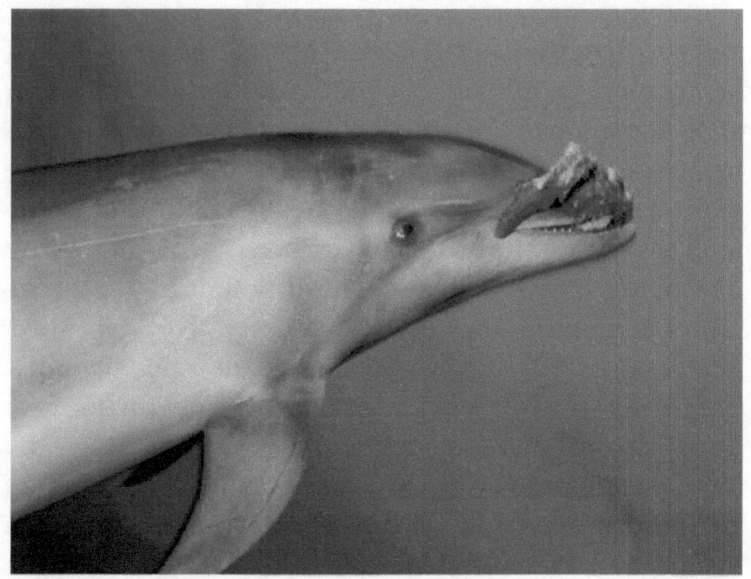

Dolphin (Tursiops aduncus) with a sponge on its snout as a tool to prevent injury when stirring up the seabed. Photo: Shutterstock

Behaviour and natural evolution
Behaviour can be defined as the internally coordinated response of living organisms (individuals or groups) to internal or external stimuli. Everything we observe about an individual or group is called behaviour. Behaviour is the chest-thumping of a silverback gorilla, the teasing of young chimpanzees, or the greeting of a new infant in the group by other group members. Doing nothing, or not responding to a stimulus, is also 'behaviour'. An organism cannot 'not behave' in response to its environment.

Behaviour can be innate or learned. Behaviour is always dependent on the context, that is, history, learning processes, the current situation and species-specific characteristics (DNA). Behaviour can change over time, sometimes slowly and sometimes very quickly, influenced by different causes. In other words, behaviour is constantly evolving. The slowest form of behavioural change is through the natural evolution of the species. A change in body shape through natural evolution will eventually lead to a change in behaviour. Just think of the finches that Darwin found on the various Galapagos Islands. When the beak of a finch changed, the finch opened seeds in a different way.

Behaviour and learning processes
Learning is a continuous process of behavioural change based on experience. In all mammals, and perhaps even all animals, the learning of behaviour changes. Learning processes follow a cyclical pattern of behaviour, perception, internal evaluation and then (new) behaviour. As long as there is no need, behaviour patterns will not change. When a behaviour does not lead to the desired result, another behaviour is tried. This description of the learning process may be a bit of a shortcut, so let's go into it a bit more. An animal interacts with its environment based on the behaviour it exhibits. Let's say a chimpanzee is looking for food. He has just found a tasty papaya and sits down to eat it. However, he accidentally sits

on an anthill. The ants respond by biting him. The chimpanzee experiences the bites as a very unpleasant experience and immediately gets up to investigate and moves away from the spot. He has either 'learned' that sitting on an anthill has an unpleasant consequence or that that particular spot in the forest is best avoided. If possible, the chimpanzee will avoid forest areas or anthills.

The principle of learning outlined above helps animals to recognise edible food and where to find it and to recognise and avoid predators. The ability to learn greatly increases the chances of survival.

Not all behaviour is based on learning processes. Innate behaviour is considered a reflex or instinct. Take the startle reflex, for example. The startle reflex causes an animal to freeze in a split second when it hears a sound or sees something suspicious. It is believed that the original purpose of this reflex was to protect an animal from being hit or attacked by a predator. This reflex is still present in humans and causes the sometimes hilarious, uncontrolled movements when people are startled. The diversity of behaviour based on reflexes and instincts is limited. In the process of natural selection, emotions and cognitions are more effective in the context of behaviour than instincts. Emotionally-driven and cognitively-driven behaviours strongly differentiate the behavioural palette and therefore increase the chances of survival. Animals that learn from their experiences are better able to adapt their behaviour and survive.

Behavioural change based on personal experience is important for short-term survival.

Group animals – animals that live close together – learn from each other. This is called 'social learning'. Social learning is faster and more effective compared to individual learning, especially when there are many others in the group to learn from. Through social learning, it is not necessary to rely solely on your own experience; instead, it is possible to make use of the experiences of many others.

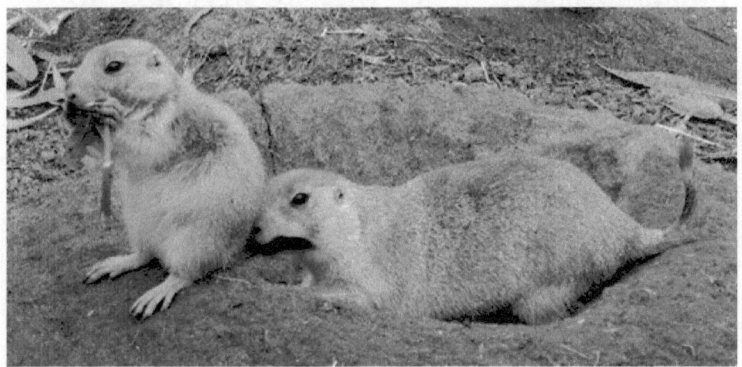

Prairie dogs (Cynomys). These funny, group-dwelling animals are known to learn by copying each other's behaviour. Photo: Jan-Paul

A good example of social learning comes from an American reintroduction project with black-tailed prairie dogs (Cynomys). Young prairie dogs raised in captivity never learn to respond to predators. A special training program was set up to teach the young prairie dogs this essential survival skill. Training sessions were carried out with and without the presence of an experienced adult prairie dog. Ultimately, prairie dogs that were trained with the experienced adult were more vigilant, sounded the alarm more often, and fled sooner than those trained without the experienced relatives. The youngsters trained with an experienced adult were also more likely to survive once released into the wild.

From social learning to cultural evolution
Culture is never rigid. Culture is fluid, constantly developing and evolving. When we think of cultural evolution, we imagine, for example, the transition of human society from the Renaissance to the Baroque. But don't fall into the trap of supposed human superiority. Animals have culture and cultural evolution, too. Let's go back to the story of macaques, who wash their carrots and potatoes before eating them. At some point, a macaque discovered that a washed carrot simply tastes better and doesn't feel gritty any longer between its teeth. Over time, other macaques adopted this behaviour through social learning. This is how the culture of washing food among macaques developed. But this is not the end of the story. Later, a monkey washing his potato discovered that biting into the potato before washing it in seawater made the potato salty and tasty and over time other monkeys imitated this behaviour. A savoury snack simply tastes better? The original culture of washing food had evolved into washing and 'seasoning' food. This is an example of cultural evolution.
Another example comes from two chimpanzee populations, one in Gombe, where primatologist Jane Goodall did her research in the 1960s, and the

other in Goualougo, Congo. It has long been known that chimpanzees use tools to catch termites. However, scientists have discovered that in Gombe, only one type of tool is used, while the chimpanzees in Goualougo use a variety of tools. Furthermore, the young apes in Goualouga learn to catch termites from their elders, while the young in Gombe are left to their own devices.

It turns out that the termites in Goualouga are much harder to catch and that different tools and training are needed to successfully outsmart the termites. By passing knowledge down from generation to generation, the technology gradually improves. This is also a form of cultural evolution. Natural behaviour based on evolution changes very slowly and is difficult to influence. Behaviour based on cultural evolution can adapt faster than natural evolution, but that does not mean it is easy to change cultural behaviour.

Pain behaviour and learning processes
Pain behaviour is a form of behaviour. As with all other behaviours, natural evolution, learning and cultural evolution apply. We have already seen that there are no major differences in the anatomy of the nervous system between mammals. It stands to reason that the influence of natural evolution on pain behaviour is therefore relatively small. In fact, some basic pain behaviours, such as withdrawing a finger from a hot flame, are probably universal among mammals. In some mammals, it is a leg or wing instead of a finger, but the response pattern is

similar. A universal, natural response to pain is to withdraw the painful body part.

In many species, learning processes and cultural evolution play a dominant role in determining variation in pain behaviour. Remember our macaques? In these monkeys, much of the pain behaviour is the result of culture more than of nature.

We must therefore be careful about what we label as 'natural' behaviour. Perhaps there is no unique natural behaviour. 'Natural' animal behaviour is more complex and diverse than we think. Learning processes and culture largely determine behaviour, including pain behaviour, not only in humans but also in many non-humans.

It would have been nice if we could compare the natural behaviour of humans and non-humans. In humans, there is actually no longer any 'natural pain behaviour'. Human pain behaviour is largely culturally determined. For a long time, we thought that animals still exhibited natural behaviour. However, this is not so self-evident. We are increasingly discovering that animals also exhibit cultural, non-natural behaviour. It is therefore no longer possible to speak of 'natural' pain behaviour in animals. And we must be very careful and reserved in our interpretation of the pain behaviour of primates, for example.

Monkeys in the wild exhibit very different pain behaviour than monkeys in captivity. The pain behaviour of monkeys in captivity is suspiciously similar to our human pain behaviour.

We can safely assume that natural evolution with regard to pain is very slow. This implies that the biological basis on which we experience pain hardly differs from that of other mammals. In humans and animal species, it has been shown that learning processes and culture influence pain behaviour. In humans, culture, through language use, has a much greater impact on pain behaviour compared to other animal species. This means that culture and cultural evolution play a decisive role in how we deal with pain.

Cultural evolution and human pain behaviour
In humans, as in all other species, there is natural evolution and cultural evolution. We have already seen that natural evolution, like our pain system, is very slow. In terms of structure, our physical pain system is no different from that of other mammals. Among humans, the neurophysiological predisposition of the pain system is the same. Differences in pain perception and pain behaviour in humans are much more the result of individual and social learning processes and culture. In other words, how we deal with pain, our perception of pain and pain behaviour are largely based on learned behaviour. So, if we want to understand something about our pain behaviour, we have to

look at what we are taught. Especially what truths are we taught?

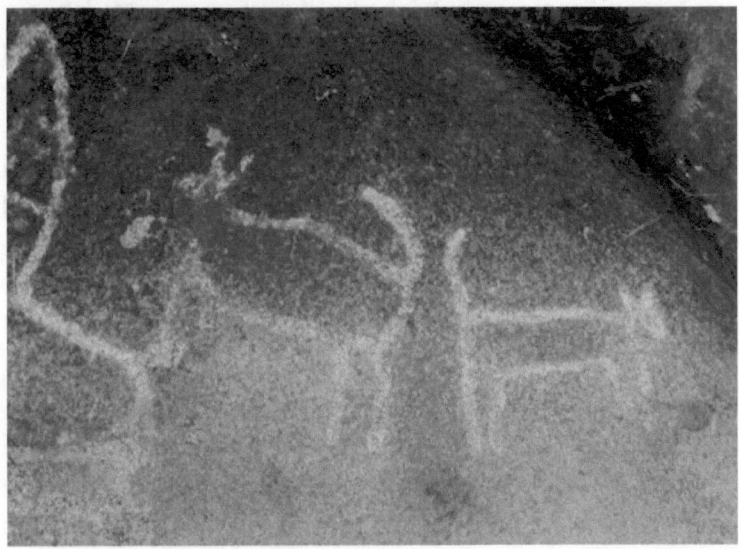

Ancient Aboriginal cave paintings from the Australian Grampians National Park over 20,000 years old. An example of the primitive figurative exchange of ideas long before the development of writing. Photo: Jan-Paul

What we learn
In the book *Sapiens*, Yuval Noah Harari describes three types of truth: the objective truth (verifiable), the subjective truth, which is subjective-personal for each individual, and the intersubjective truth. The intersubjective truth is a truth that arises when enough people believe in it.

There is less objective truth than you might think. We refer to things like gravity, time and the sun rising in the east as objective truths because they are physical laws and have been scientifically proven. Scientists like Einstein have made us realise that these truths may be true on Earth, but they may not be true throughout the universe. As a result, even these objective truths have limitations. In fact, this is true for all of science. Once we have seen a black swan, the statement, 'There are black swans', is true. But the statement, 'The Dodo is extinct', is probable but never 100% true. There is still a chance that, at some point, somewhere, a Dodo will walk out of the jungle. Declared extinction happens to various species. Like the Coelacanth, an ancient fish that was thought to have been extinct for millions of years. But somewhere in the depths of the Western Indian Ocean, the Coelacanth was found to be alive and kicking.

Subjective truth is less complicated. Subjective truth is what is consistent with your reality. So, if you think that leprechauns exist, that is your truth. A problem arises when you try to convince others that your subjective truth is actually an objective truth. It helps if there are more people who share the same opinion. If enough people are convinced of the existence of elves, it feels more and more like 'real' truth. This is what we call intersubjective truth. Intersubjective truth is a truth that arises when enough people believe in it. Intersubjective truth is therefore something completely different from the objective, 'real' truth. Intersubjective truth is not so much what is objectively 'true' but what a substantial number of people are convinced of.

A good current example is the opinion that exists that our intervertebral disc can tear if we bend forward incorrectly. Alf Nachemson, a Swedish orthopaedic surgeon, did scientific research to examine the load on the intervertebral disc in the mid-20th century. The intervertebral disc is a relatively soft structure that can be found between two consecutive vertebrae.

A few decades before Nachemson's research, it had been discovered that the outer edge of the intervertebral disc could break down. This process causes the soft inner core of the disc to be pushed outward, often into the nerve canal. This is known as a hernia nuclei pulposus (HNP), commonly referred to as a 'herniation or hernia'.

Alf Nachemson's research found that the pressure in the disc increased dramatically in certain positions. It was then assumed that this increased pressure was the cause of disc failure. The obvious conclusion was that this pressure should be avoided to prevent back injuries. In the decades that followed, experts devised and disseminated numerous lifting instructions, created ergonomic chairs, and even founded entire ergonomic consulting firms. This is a multi-million-dollar industry based on a misinterpretation of scientific research results. To this day, there are people who believe that you have to lift with a straight back to relieve pressure on the intervertebral disc. In the meantime, several new studies have shown that the intervertebral disc is perfectly capable of withstanding this changing pressure. The fact that the intervertebral disc is sometimes damaged has a completely different cause. Unfortunately, the (in this case, incorrect) intersubjective truth often wins over the objective, scientifically substantiated truth. Because there are very few truly objective truths, we often have to deal with intersubjective truths. People simply need to hold on to ideas and beliefs.

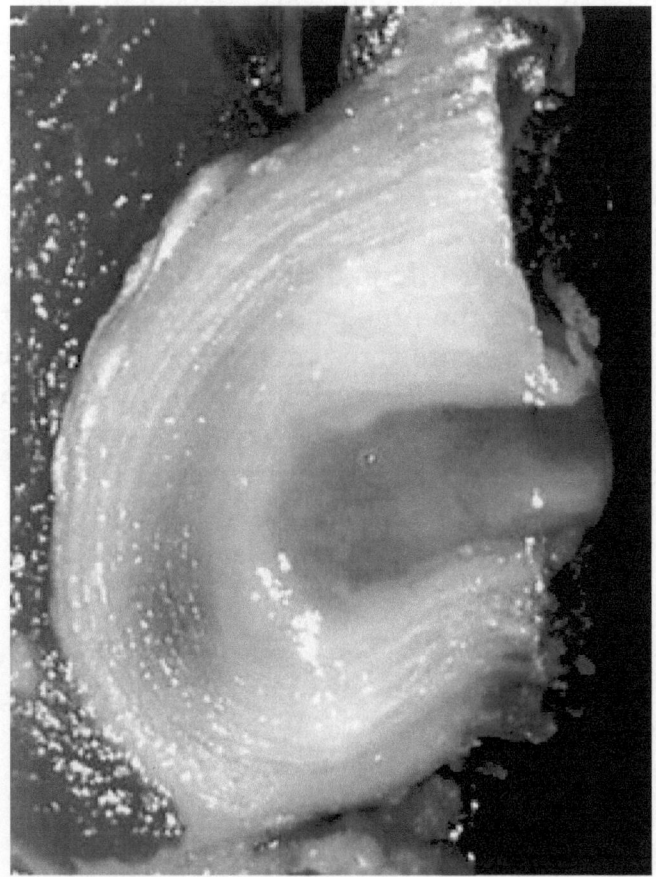

Left half of a pig intervertebral disc (Sus scrofa domesticus). Note the layers in the surrounding rim (annulus) and the soft, jelly-like core (nucleus). Photo: Jan-Paul

The problem with science and intersubjective truth
In the example of Nachemson's research into the pressure in the intervertebral discs, you might be inclined to call this a bad study. This is not the case. The research that Nachemson conducted was excellent. It is true that the pressure in the intervertebral disc can vary depending on the situation. The problem is that these pressure measurements are only one piece of the puzzle. We tend to fill in the blanks in the puzzle with our imagination or beliefs. Science itself is not the problem. The problem is that, in order to get to the full picture, we fill in the blanks between existing knowledge with interpretations and assumptions. This is one of the problems we try to show in this book. Most scientific research meets the required quality standards. How we interpret these findings is where the problem lies. We will go into this in more detail in the following chapters.

6. How Our Pain Concept Altered

'Behaviour doesn't fossilise.'
-Louis Leakey

JP: 'We're actually back in antiquity when it comes to our current view of pain.'
Vince: 'Sorry, what do you mean exactly? Why would we be back in antiquity? Haven't we made a huge development in our knowledge of our pain systems?'
JP: 'Yes, we have, but we're still going around in big circles when it comes to the general view of pain.'
Vince: 'I don't get it. If we have more knowledge, then our view will also develop, right? How can we be back in antiquity then?'
JP: 'Just wait, we'll dedicate this chapter to the scientific development and views on pain. Let's see where we end up.'
Vince: 'Well, I'm curious...'

Monkey Business

Pain as disease
Recently, the World Health Organization (WHO) recognised pain as a disease in its own right. To some, this may seem like a major step forward in our approach to chronic pain. In fact, this recognition sets us back thousands of years. The ancient Egyptians also considered pain to be a disease. Since those ancient Egyptians, our view of pain and pain mechanisms has developed slowly. In recent decades, however, our knowledge has developed much more rapidly. So, how is it possible that this increased knowledge leads to conclusions and interpretations that are similar to those of the ancient Egyptians? Is this really how we view pain? Could it be that we are on the wrong track? In this chapter, we follow the development of our scientific knowledge of pain and try to find out why we seem to be going in circles.

Early history
The art of healing is as old as humanity. The first real 'medical' manuscripts were not found until the ancient Greeks. A large amount of Greek knowledge came from the early Egyptians. These ancient Egyptian papyri describe recipes and prescriptions. These ancient texts show that the ancient Egyptians considered pain to be a disease in its own right. The early Greeks had a more nuanced approach and had different names for pain: odunè, pèma and algos. Odunè meant sharp localised pain, pèma stood for pain as part of fate, and finally, algos was used for physically diffuse, widespread pain.

Interestingly, in these ancient times, emotions were already considered important drivers for the experience of pain, just as we believe today. And pain was connected to suffering. But like the Egyptians, these ancient Greeks also considered pain to be an autonomous disease.

The Roman Celsus (1st century) was the author of *De Medicina*, a book on nutrition, pharmacy and surgery. He seems to have been one of the first to describe pain as one of the symptoms of inflammation: swelling (tumor), pain (dolor), heat (calor), redness (rubor). He and his Roman colleagues regarded pain not so much as a disease in itself, but as a symptom. This was a first step towards a more technical-empirical medicine in which pain is not a disease in itself but rather a symptom of disease or disorder. For the second-century Greek physician, surgeon and philosopher Claudius Galen (129–199), pain was an indication of an anatomical discontinuity or a sign of a sudden change in mental well-being.

Separation of body and mind
After the Romans, centuries passed without any significant changes in the scientific view of pain. Then, in the 17th century, this perception of pain changed quite suddenly and radically. Not only did the ideas introduced change our view of pain, they also fundamentally changed our understanding of body and mind. The brain behind these ideas was the famous French philosopher, mathematician and scientist René Descartes (1596–1650), who

published the book *Principia Philosophiae* in 1644. In this still-famous book, Descartes introduced his theory of the separation of body and mind.

The idea of mind and body as separate entities allowed Descartes to study and understand the human body without denying God's role and position. Although clever, Descartes did not succeed very well in his intention. The Christian church banned his books for a long time. Descartes' suggestion of separating body and mind has stuck with us to this day. Doctors and physical therapists as well as psychologists and psychiatrists all struggle with this artificial separation of body and mind that was invented long ago by Descartes.

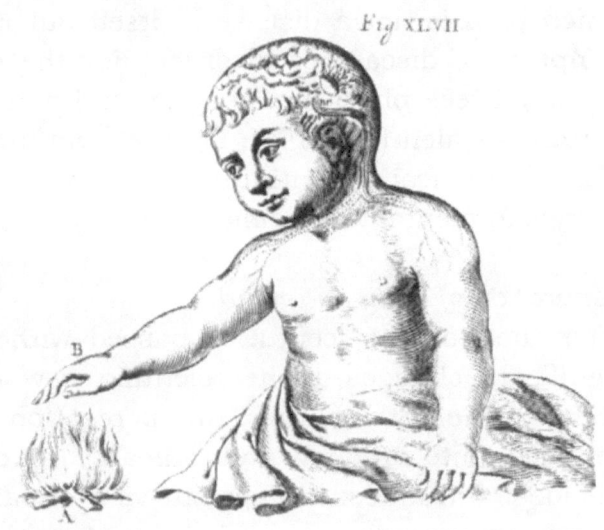

Pain consciousness visualised according to the vision of Descartes.

Pain as a technical phenomenon
After Descartes' theoretical separation of body and mind, it took several centuries before the biomedical view of pain really gained popularity. In the 19th century, German scientists advanced the knowledge of physiology, especially cell function and dysfunction (Theodor Schwann, 1810–1882, and Matthias Jakob Schleiden, 1804–1881). Physiology was assumed to be strictly mechanical. Furthermore, human functioning, both physical and psychological, was described in mechanical terms (Ernst Wilhelm Ritter von Brücke, 1819–1892, and Emil Heinrich du Bois-Reymond, 1818–1896). From this mechanical-physiological point of view, it was assumed that nociceptive stimuli were transmitted from specific receptors via nociceptive pathways to the brain. In the brain, this would lead to sensation and consciousness in humans. Pain was thought to have sensory qualities similar to touch, hearing or vision and to proceed via special conduction and perception systems. Nociceptive stimuli travel through fast-conducting A-delta nerve fibres or the slower C nerve fibres of the spinal cord. Nociceptive signals are then conducted via specific pain pathways (the spinothalamic tract) to a switching station in the thalamus. From there, the signal travels to the cortex, where sensation is supposed to occur. This view led to the idea that interrupting this conduction system could block or interrupt pain.
At the end of the 19th century, new discoveries and theories followed each other in rapid succession.

Johannes Müller (1801–1858), who studied amputees, was the first (decades before the famous Ron Melzack and Patrick Wall) to find evidence for the existence of controlling 'gates' in pain pathways. The Austrian-German physiologist Maximilian von Frey (1852–1922) already suspected that the relationship between experienced pain and the degree of stimulation is not linear. And the German neurologist Alfred Goldscheider (1858–1935) found indications for the addition of signals in the central summation. All these new findings paved the way for a completely new view of pain, which would see the light of day around the middle of the 20th century.

Beginning of the modern vision: Gate control
Around 1965, Canadian psychologist Ronald Melzack and English anatomist Patrick Wall presented a model in which pain was no longer a simple signal along a nerve pathway. They described so-called 'gates', as Johannes Müller had already done in the mid-1800s: connections between nerve pathways in the spinal cord through which pain sensations can be modulated. From that moment on, there was no way back; pain was no longer seen as a simple signal from a damaged body part to the brain but as the result of complex interactions between different parts of the body, including the brain. Melzack and Wall found that the concept of a 'gate' greatly facilitated the acceptance and popularity of the theory.

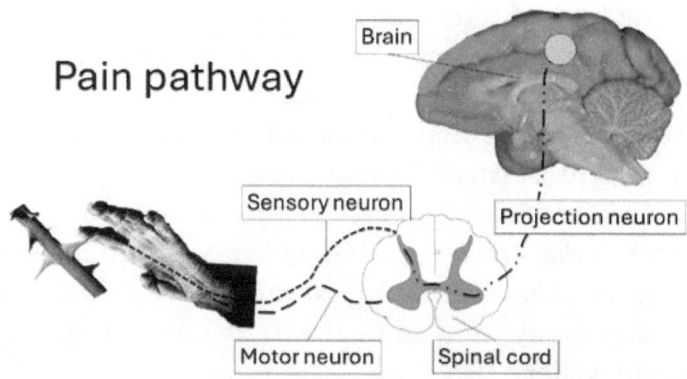

Gate control in monkey brains. The mechanism is identical to that in the human brain.

Patrick Wall recalls in an interview: 'A fortunate aspect of our 1965 publication is the use of the term "gate control". It conjures up a picture that is easy to understand, even for those who do not understand the complex physiological mechanisms on which the theory is based.'

This observation by Melzack and Wall underscores once again the importance of clever communication.

Fifty years later, this aspect of the publication still resonates. In particular, the 'gate' metaphor serves as a convenient and useful way to explain to patients what pain is and how and why it fluctuates from day to day. Many current programs for chronic pain education and pain self-management refer to the gate control theory, specifically the gate mechanism in the spinal cord.

But the idea of 'gate control' was not the end of the story. Over the years, the gate control theory has developed into the neuromatrix theory, which includes a huge amount of additional knowledge and insights. There is now much more scientific knowledge available about the phenomenon of pain. This growing knowledge has given us more insight into pain. However, understanding what pain is and, especially, how to deal with it has not exactly become easier.

Some will argue that Melzack and Wall's gate control theory was a definitive farewell to the model of Descartes. The question is whether this is really the case. Even within the gate control theory, questions such as 'Who experiences the pain?' or 'Can animals experience the emotional aspect of pain signals?' remain difficult to answer. You may wonder whether the gate control theory freed us from the perspective of Descartes. The answer is, unfortunately, 'No'. In the years that followed, the theory of pain became increasingly complex. Pain has long ceased to be the bad feeling that you want to get rid of as quickly as possible. Pain is also no longer just a protective mechanism. Pain appears to have cognitive and emotional aspects in which the brain plays a major role. And learning processes also appear to play a role in how pain is experienced. That history begins with a snail.

Pain and learning: Sensitisation
The first clue to the role of learning in relation to pain came from Eric Kandell (1927), a physician specialised in psychiatry, a neuroscientist, and a professor of biochemistry and biophysics. His research focused on learning and the nervous system. In his studies, he made extensive use of the sea snail, the Aplysia californica. The relatively simple nervous system and large neurons of this mollusc are ideal for research. Kandell discovered that repeating a painful stimulus caused the Aplysia he used to respond increasingly intensely. He also found adaptations in the nervous system of the molluscs that were related to the increased sensitivity. In line with his learning research, he discovered that he could teach the mollusc to respond defensively even to a normally neutral stimulus. Because of this increased sensitivity, Kandell used the word sensitisation in the context of learning mechanisms and memory.

Sensitisation and psychology
Another scientist who focused on learning processes and the adaptive behaviour of the brain was the German professor of neuropsychology Herta Flor (1954). She studied the close connection between physical causes and the psychological dimensions of pain. Among other things, she showed how fundamental psychological factors can contribute to the chronicity of pain. Her main findings were that learning and memory processes play an important role in the development of

chronic pain. According to Herta Flor, chronic pain is accompanied by site-specific, maladaptive, structural and functional changes in the brain. In other words, changes in the perception of the body are accompanied by pain-related learning processes.

To put it more simply, Herta Flor states that chronic pain is accompanied by structural changes in the brain, which may indicate irreversibility. According to her, such learning processes offer opportunities for new treatment methods. In the context of Herta Flor's position, it is important to note that a significant part of her research was conducted using patients with amputations. In this particular patient group, she found that mapping in the primary sensorimotor cortex changed such that input from adjacent areas occupied the area that previously received input from the now-amputated limb. These reorganizational changes were only observed in amputees with phantom pain after amputation, not in amputees without pain.

Fear-avoiding behaviour

Emotional factors have increasingly played a role in pain. As a result, psychologists and psychiatrists have become increasingly dominant in the field of pain research. Approaches to pain in which fear plays a major role are hard to miss. For example, the models of movement fear and fear avoidance. In 1990, Shashidar Kori and Robert Miller were the first to coin the term 'kinisophobia', later rewritten as *kinesiophobia*. Kori refers to the avoidance of movement or activity based on fear. This mechanism has been suggested as a central mechanism in the development of persistent back pain. The underlying idea for this model is that the fear of pain and the possibility of re-injury may be more disabling than pain itself.

Many psychologists have embraced this concept. Johan Vlaeyen, a Dutch psychologist, claims that pain provokes fear, which, when coupled with movement, can direct the focus toward movement. In other words, pain can make patients reluctant to move.

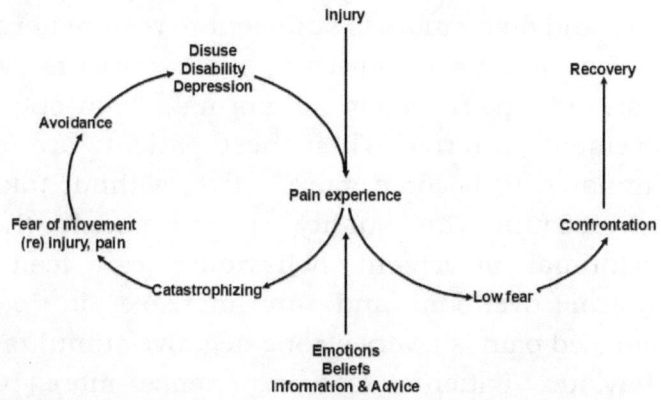

Fear-avoidance model by Vlaeyen. Graph: Johan Vlaeyen

Limited movement can lead to a decline in the patient's condition and physical capacity. This can throw the physical resilience and daily burden out of balance. And that can lead to overload and increased pain. This line of thought assumes that encouraging patients to increase their physical activity and to confront and expose their fear can help reduce their fear and allow them to recover from chronic (back) pain. This concept has two special aspects. Firstly, this approach assumes that avoiding activity is common in chronic pain. In the practice of pain rehabilitation, this is often not the case. Many patients, if not the majority of patients, remain very active despite their pain. This behaviour is at odds with the idea that patients avoid movement based on fear. The fear-avoidance model completely ignores this significant group exhibiting the opposite behaviour. Secondly, the Vlaeyen model assumes that simply becoming active and doing more is sufficient to restore normal physical function. However, most patients with persistent pain show abnormal, non-optimal movement patterns. When these patients are only stimulated to become more active, without taking into account the quality of movement, these suboptimal movement behaviours can lead to physical overload and an increase in pain. Increased pain is a very strong negative stimulus for behaviour. Patients who experience more pain during activity quickly become reluctant to be more active. Treatment methods such as Graded Exposure and Graded Activity will be particularly successful if sufficient attention is paid to the quality of movement. Unfortunately, this aspect of movement quality is rarely included in the concept of fear avoidance.

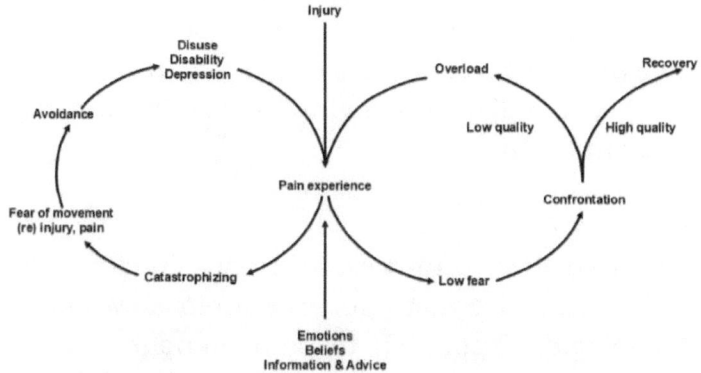

Adapted fear-avoidance model of Vlaeyen by authors. Specific behaviour is essential to get positive emotional feedback. Low quality causes more pain and a negative response. High-quality movement behaviour causes a positive response (reduction in pain). Graph: Jan-Paul.

Pain under control
By the end of the 20th century, the dominant psychological approach to (chronic) pain had stimulated the development of all kinds of behavioural treatment protocols, such as cognitive behavioural therapy (CBT) and acceptance-commitment therapy (ACT). One of the first authors to write about these concepts in the Netherlands was Frits Winter in his book *'Pain under control'* (Original Dutch title: *'Pijn de baas'*). The message underlying his approach is: 'Do not strive to get rid of your pain, but ask yourself, *how can I, despite my pain, live a valuable life?*' When you manage to be active with sufficient relaxation, the pain becomes bearable. Reducing pain is not the main goal but an automatic consequence of the changed movement

behaviour. Unspoken in this approach is the premise that physical recovery is not an option. By choosing the psychological or behavioural path, the therapeutic effect lies mainly in the mind and no longer in the body.

Explain pain
The Australian authors, scientist-clinician David Butler and neuroscientist Lorimer Moseley, take the psychological approach to pain management to a new level. In their remarkable book, *Explain Pain*, they present simple, accessible concepts about pain. Their starting point is that the more we understand our pain, the less it will bother us. According to them, pain is an experience constructed in response to dangers and threats in our bodies. This response is influenced by our thoughts, beliefs and context. Knowledge about these mechanisms is therefore the key to managing your pain.
Butler and Moseley's book is a good, detailed reflection of our current view of pain. In their view, neurophysiology, psychology and emotions are of primary importance for understanding pain. The body is seen merely as a vehicle that needs special instructions on how to behave in order to move with as little pain as possible.

Our modern pain perspective
As this chapter describes, we have come a long way in understanding pain. We have also come a long way in understanding the underlying mechanisms

and techniques to suppress pain. Despite all this knowledge, millions of people today suffer from chronic pain. Some of these people suffer from specific diseases such as cancer or physical conditions such as amputations. In the latter group, there are specific and unavoidable circumstances in which pain is an unwanted secondary effect. Technical solutions such as medication, injections, neurostimulation and surgical intervention or behavioural approaches such as meditation and cognitive training are indispensable when dealing with such pain.

In addition to these relatively well-defined situations, there is an ocean of poorly understood chronic pain conditions such as back pain, headaches, fibromyalgia and CSSD (Chronic Somatic Symptom Disorder) or PSS (Persistent Somatic Symptoms). For these patients, there are two main paths that can be followed. One is to chemically or mechanically interrupt the pathway that leads to pain sensations. This solution follows the more biomedical view of pain, where general practitioners, anaesthetists or neurologists prescribe medication, neurostimulation or surgical interventions such as cutting or burning nerves. The other is to find a way to deal with the pain mentally. Psychologists, psychiatrists and rehabilitation clinics advocate this approach. In both directions, the physical aspects are consistently ignored.

In 2017, the World Health Organization (WHO), the global body that sets standards for health policy, proposed a new definition of 'chronic pain' that they believed 'could significantly improve the care of patients with persistent pain'. They expected that classifying chronic primary pain as a disease would lead to a renewed interest in pain and how health systems assess and treat it. We must realise, however, that by taking this global step, we are taking a step back, as we have seen before, to the ancient Egyptians and Greeks who considered pain to be a disease. So what are the implications for how we deal with pain?

7. How We Deal with Pain

'Reality is created by the mind. We can change our reality by changing our mind.'
- *Plato*

Vince: 'So that's how our knowledge of pain has developed over the centuries?'
JP: 'Yes, indeed.'
Vince: 'But even now that we know so much, we are still not able to cure all forms of pain.'
JP: 'Yes, unfortunately, that is the case.'
Vince: 'Oh, that's nice (cynical tone). Do we have any idea why?'
JP: 'Well, no, but maybe we should look at how people deal with their pain today.'
Vince: 'Good idea; maybe we can find a clue as to what's wrong and how it can be improved.'
JP: 'Yes, but we have to keep in mind that it is utopian to think that we can relieve every form of pain.'

Do something about it!
Since ancient times, our perception of pain has changed considerably. Scientific perspectives are slowly seeping into our daily ideas and thoughts about pain. Slowly but surely, our perception of pain is shifting from a one-to-one relationship with damage to pain resulting from a complex interplay of different factors. We understand that emotions also play a role in how we experience pain. Some even assume that there is such a thing as mental pain. This is pain that we do indeed experience, but it has a mental cause.

If our knowledge of pain has developed over time, does that mean that we also have less pain? Unfortunately, this is not the case. Studies among different population groups show that more and more people suffer from one form of pain or another. This trend is visible not only in the Netherlands but also throughout the Western world. Pain is one of our greatest medical challenges. Despite all efforts, more and more healthcare money is spent on pain management every year.

How is it possible that, despite all the developments in the field of pain management, pain seems to occur more often? The gradual increase in the average age of our population may be an important factor. As you get older, the chance of physical complaints and pain increases. At least, that is what is often assumed. Lifestyle and environment are increasingly recognised as determinants of a long and healthy life. But there are countless young people who also experience pain and even in this group of young people the pain does not seem to decrease.

Can we explain why our experience of pain, in general, does not seem to decrease but actually increases? Could it be that our increased knowledge about pain is counterproductive? That it serves not to reduce pain but actually worsens it? This may seem contradictory, so let us take a closer look at this idea. To do this, we need to examine our general world perspective.

The malleable world
For centuries, humanity has shaped the world to its will and we are very good at it. Since the first mud hut we have built skyscrapers hundreds of meters high. Since the first potato was planted we have grown megatons of food. We have conquered the sea, turned the sea into land or brought water to where there is a drought. We have been very successful in this. However, this success is going to our heads. We believe that the current global warming is caused by man. We also think that we, as humanity, can slow down or even stop global warming. This is not about whether or not man is the cause of global warming. It is about believing that we can do something about it. That it is feasible. That we have the ability to influence the climate on an enormous, global scale. And whether or not we succeed in this says something about the image we have of ourselves. It reflects the extent to which we believe that we have the power to shape and control the world around us. And the way we

view the controllability of our environment also has an effect on the way we view our physical well-being.

The malleable body
As long as we have existed, we have struggled with physical discomfort. In addition to pain, we also have to deal with other physical discomforts such as constipation, inflammation, vermin, scabies, itching, irritated skin, fungi and much more. For as long as we've known, people have been looking for solutions to these discomforts. And that does not only apply to people. We are increasingly aware of how animals also strive to alleviate their discomforts. It is known that dogs eat grass when they are nauseous. Chimpanzees in the wild that suffer from malaria specifically search for and eat certain minerals in the soil, which they normally do not do. Or they eat certain bitter leaves to rid their intestines of worms (nematodes). Self-medication in animals is not at all unusual. For example, some birds rub ants on their bodies. The formic acid produced by the ants works as a fungicide or bactericide. Capuchin monkeys also rub their fur with plants that have anti-insect properties. And it goes further. Orangutans (Pongo Pygmaeus) in Borneo sometimes eat plants (Dracaena Cantleyi) with anti-inflammatory properties. Whether it is birds, bees, lizards or elephants, they all engage in forms of self-medication. When it comes to medicine, humans, with their immense

pharmaceutical industry, are, of course, the best at self-medicating.

Our urge to control discomfort and limitations goes beyond medication alone. Technological developments make it possible to renew body joints and even internal organs. Think of replacing hips, knees and shoulders or transplanting organs such as the heart, lungs, kidneys and liver. These types of interventions allow us to function better and even postpone death. And it doesn't stop there. Instead of finding satisfaction in these possibilities, people assume that these techniques not only guarantee survival but also improve their quality of life. In addition to avoiding life-threatening conditions, there is also the desire to achieve non-life-threatening desirable improvements. Wrinkles are smoothed out with Botox injections. The size and shape of numerous body parts are adjusted at will. Breasts, buttocks and calves are shaped according to what is desirable, using bags of silicone, saline or body fat. In short, our body is increasingly seen as a malleable, adaptable and, above all, manufacturable utensil.

Our malleable pain
Pain, like many other aspects of life, must be manageable. Who hasn't seen the commercial with a charming grey-haired model playing his daily game of tennis with a face contorted in pain. Until the painkilling cream brings relief! The message is that even as you get older, you don't have to

accept pain. We (says the manufacturer of the cream) can

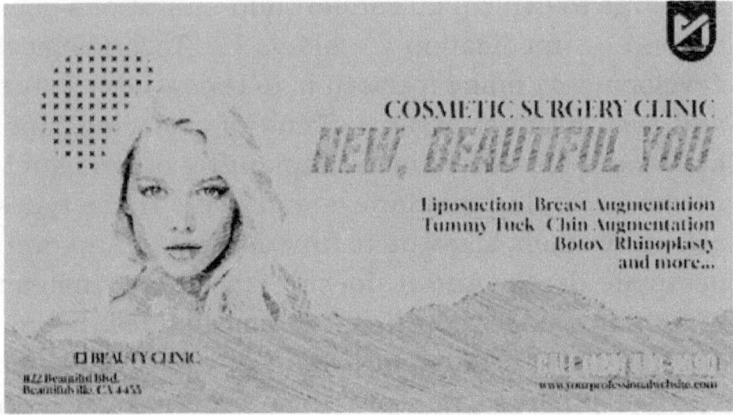

Plastic surgery suggests the idea of a body that can be shaped. Unfortunately, this is a misconception. Advertisement from the internet.

take away the pain for you. This message – that pain doesn't have to be there – gets through everywhere. Until about forty years ago, dentists drilled holes in teeth without anaesthesia. Anaesthesia was only administered for more serious procedures. In time, the dentist started asking if anaesthesia was needed at the first groan. Now, even for the smallest cavity, they use anaesthetics.

Before you know it, you get a temporary blockage of the nerve pathways in the jaw area. The result is that hours after the treatment, you still spill coffee or, worse, bite your lower lip uncontrollably until it bleeds. We want to be able to live our lives without pain. Pain is so annoying and disruptive that we want to banish it from our lives completely. And that does not only apply to physical pain.

Mental pain, sadness
In addition to physical pain, humans can also suffer from mentally induced pain. As far as we know, mentally induced pain has not yet been scientifically proven in animals. Although there might be indications. There are very different forms of mental pain. Think of heartbreak or the pain you feel when losing a loved one. These kinds of feelings are not only reserved for humans. In elephants and chimpanzees, when a member of their species is lost, behaviour is seen, that seems to indicate feelings of mourning. However, we do not know exactly what these animals experience, but we do not know that about our fellow human beings either. Such feelings are very personal experiences of a type which we can never really know how it feels for someone else. At most, we can imagine how we would experience a similar sensation ourselves and assume that it is the same for the other person. It remains a personal, subjective experience. This applies to humans and animals.

If you were to look at the family tree of people at the beginning of the 20th century, you would come across something terrible. Most of these people had a large number of children, but many of these children died prematurely. Losing a child is considered one of the most terrible forms of loss. Such losses have a great impact on parents in our society.

Our contemporary society prepares for such a trauma by setting up social workers and agencies where parents who experience such a trauma can seek help. If the loss of one child is a great trauma, imagine what people had to go through at the beginning of the 20th century. They would lose not one but several children. That must have been a tragic, incomprehensibly great loss. One wonders how these people were able to continue their lives. Or is something else going on here? Could it be that the death of children at the beginning of the 20th century, although incredibly sad, was just something that happened at that time? That you, as a parent, knew that this could happen to you?

Could it be that in our current, controllable society, the death of a child is not only terrible but also unacceptable at the same time? After all, everything in our society must be manageable. It is our expectation that such a loss can be prevented. This implies that, although the loss of a child is always devastating, people in the early 20th century may have dealt with it differently than we do today. Because expectations are changing. We increasingly see the world as something we can shape and control. When life doesn't unfold as we expect, the impact is more intense. If we expect to be able to prevent things from happening we become more sensitive to them when they do happen.

Mental pain, social interaction
A similar but less severe example of this mechanism is the unpleasant feeling that arises when we feel hurt, insulted, ignored or ridiculed. Nowadays, people in our Western society are becoming increasingly sensitive to forms of insult or unfair treatment. Think of Donald Duck comics or Roald Dahl books that are rewritten because certain passages may be offensive. Here, we have the curious phenomenon that the more we avoid or remove potentially offensive things, the more sensitive we seem to become to them.

The absence of negative stimuli increases the body's sensitivity to them. This is standard neurophysiology: when you enter a quiet room, your hearing becomes more sensitive, and in the dark, your eyes become more sensitive to light. In many cases, a reduction in certain stimuli makes us more sensitive to them. Therefore, there is a downside to the growing emphasis on socio-political correctness and the elimination or avoidance of potentially offensive expressions. Increasing our sensitivity to negatively labelled interactions in any form does not seem to be a good development. This is not a licence to insult, taunt, or discriminate against fellow human beings, but it should make us think about keeping our brains healthy. To keep our bodies healthy, we are advised to engage in regular physical activity. Perhaps, to keep our brains resilient, we need to be regularly taunted or mocked or experience a measured loss.

The pain of not having control
The way we humans think about pain secretly contains a double layer. It starts with the pain that you can experience. In this basic experience, we are no different from other animals. If the pain persists, we start to suffer from it. The idea that this suffering is a typical human characteristic is outdated. Watch the videos of the animal protection fund. Images are shown of abused donkeys or bears. They are malnourished, with skin lesions and other injuries. You can see it in their eyes: the animal is suffering. It is often said that we cannot know this. After all, the animal does not express its pain in words. Yet the non-verbal communication is enough for us to realise that the animal is suffering. Just as we experience it with other animals. We do not imagine this. It is becoming increasingly clear that suffering and also emotions in general can be inferred from facial expressions. Research into this is still in its infancy, but it is promising.

But there is a pitfall: we live with the illusion that the world around us can be controlled. That imperfections or discomforts can be brushed away. And that belief also applies to pain. The fact that, contrary to our expectations, we are not in control makes our problem bigger. We are in pain. We are bothered by it. And then we suffer from the fact that we are not in control. We have lost control. This idea undermines our fundamental sense of control over our lives, over our existence. This suffering about suffering is caused by our misplaced idea of control over life. This level of suffering is probably something that people bring upon themselves. It is not clear whether this is a human or, for example, a culture-bound phenomenon. It depends on the extent to which the individual feels that he or she has control over life. This aspect varies greatly between cultures. In any case, as far as we know, it does not occur in animals.

Control pain
From the perspective of the controllable world, we also accept less and less that we sometimes experience pain, both physically and mentally. For severe pain, such as during surgical interventions, this is quite understandable. Regardless of the experience of the victim, the surgeon and the outcome of the operation benefit when the person being operated on remains immobile. The introduction of ether anaesthesia around 1846 at Massachusetts General Hospital, which made the first completely painless operation possible, was a real milestone. Today, there are very diverse forms of pain management. These range from commonly available simple painkillers to major procedures designed to permanently interrupt pain. We will take a closer look at some of these methods. In order to tackle pain in cancer patients worldwide, the WHO developed the pain ladder in 1986. Today, this pain ladder is also used to treat other types of pain.

Simple discomforts (Step 1 on the WHO pain ladder)
Almost everyone can experience pain at some point. Pain can manifest as muscle pain, headache or toothache. Every year, millions of simple painkillers such as aspirin and paracetamol or non-steroidal anti-inflammatory drugs (NSAIDs such as ibuprofen and diclofenac) are sold. Most of these drugs inhibit the production of substances that increase stimuli to the nervous system. Because fewer stimuli pass through, the pain decreases. Although these drugs are available without a prescription, they are not without danger. With continued use, the risk of stomach and intestinal complaints, closing of the trachea and stomach bleeding is not unlikely.

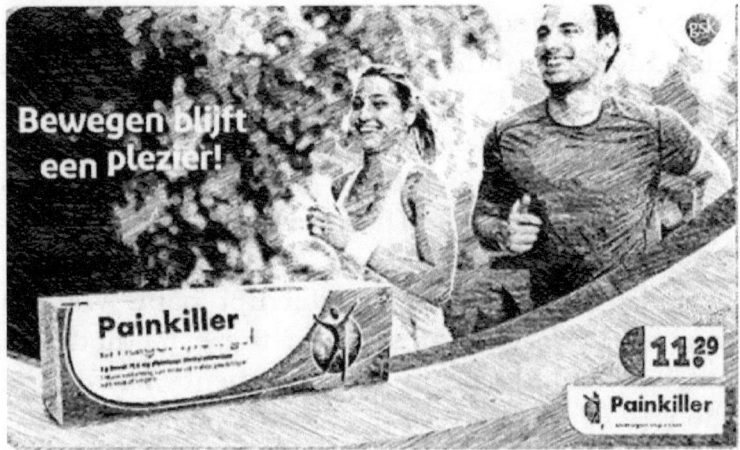

Advertisement for pain relief ointment. Gives the impression that you can control your pain and continue with your activities. Advertisement from the internet.

Heavy stuff (Steps 2 and 3 on the WHO pain ladder)
If the relatively simple drugs do not work, stronger drugs such as tramadol, morphine, fentanyl and oxycodone are available on prescription. These drugs belong to the group of strong to very strong painkillers. In contrast to the previous group, these drugs do not work peripherally but rather in the central nervous system, where they inhibit the sensation of pain. These drugs do not have an anti-inflammatory effect. These drugs belong to the class of opioids, which means that their use can lead to tolerance and even addiction.

Next level: 'Burn the place down'
If even the stronger opioids don't work, the options become scarce. For example, it is possible to inject opioids directly into the nervous system. But we can't go much further than that. We then move on to more destructive methods, such as burning off nerve branches that are thought to contribute to the persistent pain signals. We've come up with complicated terms like coagulation, a process that basically involves burning off a part of a nerve branch. On closer inspection, this process seems rather peculiar. Despite the technical sophistication of the methods used, they ultimately amount to destruction or removal. And from that perspective, our way of doing things still seems rather primitive. It is like the dog that is inclined to bite off its own leg when it is caught in a trap. And even these rather aggressive methods are sometimes not enough to provide relief. Some of these patients are

still in pain. At this point, there are only a few options left.

Let's talk about it

When all else fails, we move on to non-physical pain treatments. That's a fancy way of saying, 'we can't help you physically, so let's talk about it'. We are now entering a new and somewhat obscure field of pain therapy. This type of treatment no longer focuses on the pain itself but instead focuses on the impact of the pain on the patient's life. Although it is called 'pain treatment', the pain itself is not really addressed at this stage.

These psychological treatments include behavioural control, depression treatment, acceptance treatments or other forms of psychological treatment. The goal is to help the patient resume their life as best they can despite the pain. This is akin to a psychic lobotomy, as Damasio described in his book, *I Feel, Therefore I Am*. A patient with persistent pain after a lobotomy/brain injury still had the same amount of pain but was no longer bothered by it. Accepting that there is pain can help to reduce suffering. It is a possibility, but it poses a considerable challenge for people suffering from chronic pain: 'Accept that the pain is there. There is no other choice than to embrace this idea and let it go.' The essence of pain is to be acknowledged, seen and heard. This letting go and accepting is a huge challenge. Some patients who follow this form of treatment manage to pick up their lives again despite their pain. Some even experience less pain.

For others, this form of treatment is a poor alternative without giving a real solution. There are many studies in scientific literature that show positive results with this behavioural approach compared to other current treatments. One wonders whether the apparent optimism is based on these results or whether the results of the treatments against which they are compared are even worse.

Relation with pain
So, this is where we are now. Scientifically, we understand much more about the neurophysiological mechanisms behind pain. We have developed numerous tools and techniques to control, suppress or eliminate pain. The fact that we do not have to feel pain when visiting a dentist or during a surgical procedure makes life a lot more pleasant for us.

At the same time, the enormous and still growing number of people with (persistent) pain shows us how poorly we have succeeded in eradicating pain. In fact, it seems that the pain we try to suppress only comes back more intensely. This is not how we imagine our controllable world should be.

Perhaps we are making a mistake in our thinking. We need to better realise that pain simply does not conform to the rules of our controllable world. Pain has a function that we cannot ignore. Pain is of great importance and not just an unpleasant feeling.

Perhaps our intersubjective truth is further removed from objective truth than we think. Let us go back to the function of pain. We now have a clear understanding of the neurophysiological principles of pain. What is the purpose or use of pain?

8. The Purpose of Pain

'Great is the power of steady misrepresentation, but the history of science shows that fortunately this power does not long endure.'
-*Charles Darwin*

Vince: 'What's the point of all this anyway?'
JP: 'You mean of life? That's a big question...'
Vince: 'No, I mean of pain. What's the purpose of it? Why can't we just have protective reflexes without this annoying experience we call pain?'
JP: 'Well, some people do enjoy experiencing pain...'
Vince: 'Yeah, but that's not what I mean. I mean "normal" people and animals. Why do they have to go through something they want to avoid?'
JP: 'Exactly because of that.'
Vince: 'Because of what exactly?'
JP: 'The fact that they want to avoid pain is exactly why there's pain in the first place.'
Vince: 'Oh boy, I feel another chapter coming on.'
JP: 'Yeah, let's look at what the purpose of pain actually is.'

Where there's smoke...
While on holiday, I (JP) got a call from my neighbour. An alarm had gone off in our house. Luckily, our good neighbour had our house key and she was able to enter our property. One of those round detectors on the ceiling was the source of the noise. After the neighbour checked the house twice and found nothing alarming, she removed the detector from the ceiling and took out the battery, after which peace returned.

The following week, when I got home, I put the battery back in the detector. No alarm. But as soon as I took a shower, the detector went off again. Concerned, we turned off the boiler and called a repairman. After two days of cold showers, the repairman finally arrived. He quickly concluded that there was nothing wrong with the boiler. The detector turned out to be a smoke detector, not a carbon monoxide detector. In the end, the smoke detector itself turned out to be defective and not working properly.

What is the moral of this story? Firstly, it is possible for an alarm system to malfunction and trigger an incorrect alarm. Consider the sensitisation of the nervous system, as discussed in detail in Chapter 4.

Secondly, when an alarm goes off, it is wise to first assume that a possible calamity is taking place and to look for possible danger. This is exactly the same with pain.

When we are in pain, we want to know what is going on with our body. Figuring out what is causing an alarm can be difficult. This is also very similar to pain. With many of our pain experiences, we cannot figure out what is physically causing the pain.

> Vince: 'Why did we have to come up with a mechanical example here? We were just looking at all kinds of examples in humans and animals...'
>
> JP: 'You're right, Vince, but it was hard to find a biological example of something breaking down.'
>
> Vince: 'I can imagine that, but there are also examples like rheumatoid arthritis or allergies. In those cases, biological systems get disrupted.'
>
> JP: 'Yes, damn, you're right! It can indeed happen in biological systems. But do you mind if we stick to the mechanical example? It's a handy story in relation to pain. And it really happened!'
>
> Vince: 'Well, okay, I'll let you get away with it this time!'

False alarm
Yes, it can happen. A false alarm as a result of a defective system. We are mainly talking about poor quality products from unreliable manufacturers from a vague and far-off country. But it would be unrealistic to claim that our bodies were made by an unreliable manufacturer. Our pain system has developed over millions of years. Design flaws in the pain system are likely to have gradually

diminished and our neurophysiological system is very refined. As a result, it is not likely to be prone to errors. But to be fair, there is always a small possibility that our pain system will become disrupted. But would such a form of disruption apply to millions of people worldwide? A product with such a margin of error would have been taken off the market long ago. Although it is not impossible, a defective pain system is not the most obvious reason for persistent pain. But what are the more obvious reasons why pain persists?

Why raise the alarm
According to the definition of pain, the most obvious cause of pain is tissue damage or the threat of tissue damage. This is also the most common reason why we feel pain. And when we feel pain, our first reaction is to investigate what is causing this discomfort. We are not alone in this. Primates are known to want to know what is happening to their bodies. For example, they use a mirror or reflection in water to inspect their teeth or other body parts that are difficult to see. We humans go much further. We have developed all kinds of techniques to assess how our body is functioning and to detect abnormalities.

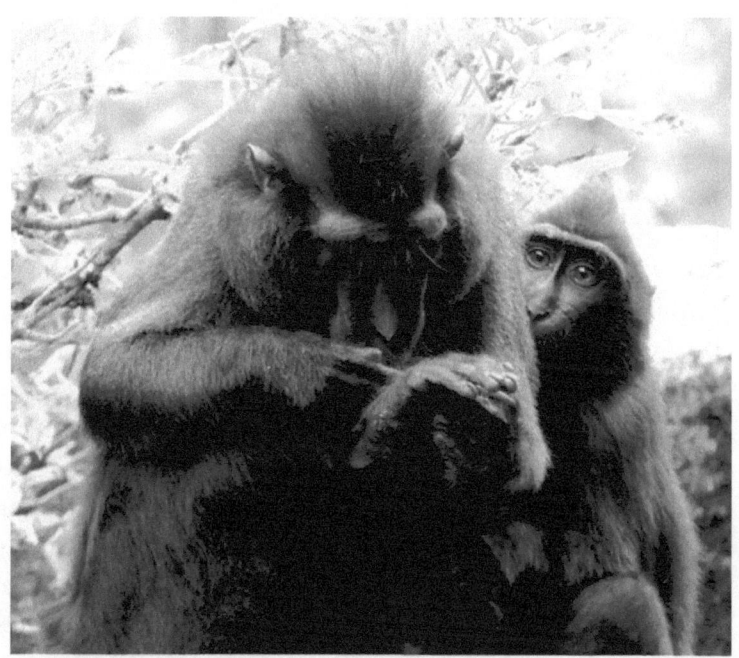

Black or crested macaque (Macaca nigra) inspecting its wounded foot, closely watched by one of its comrades. Photo: Jan-Paul

We use a stethoscope to listen to sounds coming from our body. We also have tools to look into the various openings in our body. With endoscopes, we can go even further inside. With these endoscopes, we can reach normally inaccessible places in our body through artificial holes (incisions). There are imaging techniques such as ultrasound, x-rays, MRI and CT scans.
With all these advanced analytical possibilities, we are able to examine our body for abnormalities. These abnormalities can explain our pain. Because if you find an abnormality, you may be able to do

something about it. It may lead you to the cause of the pain.

Pain relief
If something is found that is believed to be causing the pain then of course, we want to do something about it. Don't overestimate our therapeutic capabilities! There are chemicals that have pain-relieving properties. We have a number of electrical stimuli that can suppress pain signals. We have the possibility of technically advanced surgical interventions, some even using surgical robots. But in fact, all these interventions come down to sewing or stapling, sealing, removing or cauterizing. This is not very different from what was done in the Middle Ages. Of course, it is technically much more advanced and subtle and the possibility of anaesthesia makes a huge difference compared to the Middle Ages. Often with these interventions, we can help the patient resolve the issue and ultimately reduce pain. Strangely enough, in a large number of cases, pain does not seem to disappear. In fact, pain often returns after some time, sometimes worse than before the operation. Do we have an explanation for this?

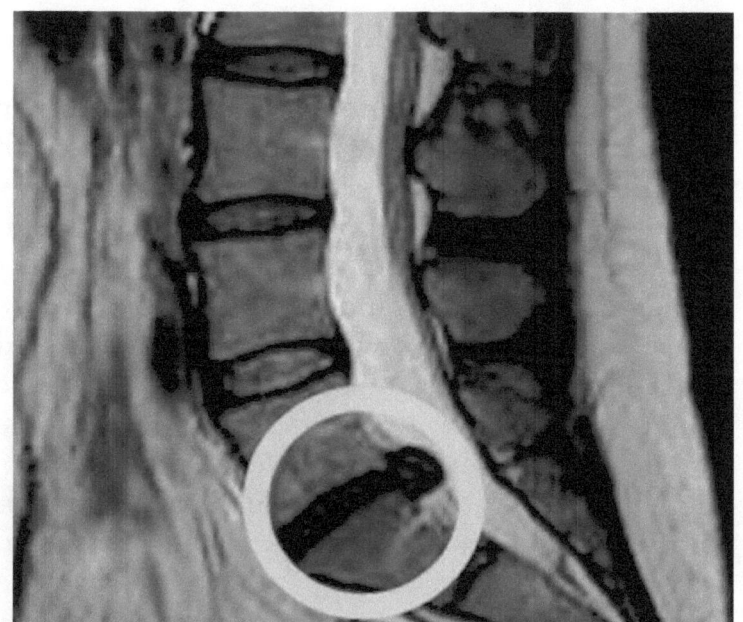

Scan of a lower back with a circled hernia inter-vertebral disc. The round structure takes up space in the white area (cauda equina, distal aspect of spinal cord). Photo: Anonymous

Persisting Pain

We have a fairly simple view of our body: if we have pain and find something strange that shouldn't be there, we remove it. In the case of a splinter in your finger, this is perfectly logical. We assume that when the splinter is gone, the pain will also go away. This is exactly the same idea we have in regard to the countless hernia operations that are performed each year on people with back problems. This is how it works. Let's assume that someone is experiencing back pain and pain in their lower leg. This may be accompanied by changes in the sensation in the leg or even loss of muscle function.

Monkey Business

Clinical assessment and imaging (scans) confirm whether there is a hernia in the back. Such a hernia can press on the nerve branches coming out of the spinal column. The material that has come out of the intervertebral disc causes an inflammatory reaction and also produces a temporary increase in pressure at the back of the spinal canal. The inflammatory reaction and the increased pressure cause the specific symptoms: pain, altered sensation, numbness and sometimes loss of muscle function. A frequently chosen solution is the surgical removal of the bulging core material. This normalises the pressure, reduces the inflammation and allows the back to recover. It is obvious to assume that this procedure will also relieve the pain. It is also not unusual for the pain and other symptoms to decrease after this operation. Stranger still is that, in many cases, the pain persists or returns after some time. In such cases, the image of what is happening in our body does not correspond to reality. We thought that the operation would solve the problem, but that does not happen: the pain remains. The disappointed surgeon will want to know whether he performed the operation correctly. He checks whether the surgical wounds have healed properly and whether there are adhesions in the scar tissue. It is not uncommon for a repeat operation to be proposed.

What we must remember here is that this process is mainly about looking for explanations for the persistent pain from a structural perspective. If we do not find a structural cause, we will quickly run out of options. A popular solution today is to switch to the model of the dysregulated nervous system. 'Dear Sir or Madam, you have already had so much trouble with your back that it has become oversensitive (sensitised), and with the stress and frustration about your back and worries about your career, you are focussing on your nervous system and making the situation worse.'

All things considered, it is quite amazing how easily and seemingly without slightest hesitation we switch from structural thinking to neurophysiological thinking.

Acute pain versus chronic pain
In the world of pain, we distinguish between acute and chronic pain. We label pain as 'chronic' if it lasts for a longer period of time, usually longer than 6 weeks or 3 months. The reasoning behind this time frame is that this is the average time that damaged tissue needs to recover. It is a somewhat simplistic and maybe even naive assumption that if tissue has had sufficient recovery time, tissue damage can no longer be a reason for pain. So there must be causes other than tissue damage when pain is still present. Those causes would then have to do with a dysregulation of the nervous system. But the distinction between acute and chronic pain is more complex. Since it is assumed that chronic pain is related to dysregulation of the nervous system, it is, as a 'logical' consequence, also assumed that psychological and social factors play an important role in our pain. In acute pain, the

influence of psychological and social factors is considered much less prominent. As if someone does not worry about acute pain or the environment cannot react strongly to an acute problem. Some authors claim that psychosocial factors become more dominant in chronic pain. It is unclear whether this is really the case.

(Imminent) damage and pain
According to the prevailing theories, pain occurs as a reaction to tissue damage or impending tissue damage. If there is no damage, there is no pain. In the case of impending tissue damage, the nervous system also reacts and pain can occur. In the case of actual damage, (more) pain occurs, which decreases again during the recovery process. This concept cannot explain persistent (chronic) pain. For this, we are forced to turn to the sensitisation theory, which assumes that the central nervous system is disrupted.

An important question that arises but is rarely asked is: how can the nervous system become disrupted without any apparent reason or cause? This question has not yet been satisfactorily answered in science, although it has been suggested that, for example, stress and uncertainty can be driving factors.

In order to better understand the underlying mechanisms of sensitisation, we would like to briefly describe our experiences with a large group of chronic patients with back and pelvic girdle pain.
Pain reduction through behavioural change

The Spine & Joint Centre is a Dutch outpatient rehabilitation centre that treats patients with chronic back pain. Since its establishment in 1996, more than 15,000 people have been treated. The people who come here have had pain for many years on average. Most of them have received various other treatments, usually with limited results. That is why most of these patients are considered 'therapy-resistant'. An important first part of the Spine & Joint Centre programme is that patients take rest periods. They have to lie down for fifteen minutes every 1 or 2 hours to relax the body. The vast majority of patients experience a clear reduction in their pain within a few days, provided that they apply these rest periods properly. According to supporters of the sensitisation theory, this rapid effect on pain should not be possible. After all, central sensitisation is the result of structural changes in the central nervous system. This is not expected to change in such a short time. Could there be another explanation for this exceptionally rapid and clinically relevant reduction in pain? This change in behaviour, that is, taking these moments of rest, is not the complete treatment but a condition to be able to work on sustainable recovery and reduction of pain. Taking moments of rest and relaxing muscle tension is an important first step to calming the pain in a sustainable way.

Sore Muscles after a workout
Another phenomenon that many people will recognise is the pain and stiffness in their muscles after intensive activity, workout or sports. This pain can last for several days and be severe. We assume that waste products in the muscles and the process of muscle building cause this pain, not muscle damage itself. So, it seems very likely that there is a third phase in which pain can occur. Not only with (1) tissue damage or (2) impending tissue damage but also with (3) the body's perception that there is a suboptimal physical situation. A situation that could ultimately also lead to tissue damage. If a body does not function sufficiently in balance, the nervous system can cause pain before there is even a threat of tissue damage. This is to indicate that the physical situation is potentially threatening.

Protection
The fundamental function of pain is to protect and this protection may be much more subtle than just protection against (imminent) tissue damage. Our nervous system is extremely advanced. It not only responds to immediate or imminent tissue damage but also to damage that could possibly occur. The nervous system can send a signal that the body is not in an optimal condition. The body is working 'out of balance'. Our body can send (pain) signals to let us know that something is 'not right' without tissue damage or even imminent tissue damage. At a stage where we can apparently still do everything,

pain is already occurring, even though we are apparently not limited by real physical problems.

Pain as a trigger for behavioural change
Why would we stop our activities when we can apparently do everything physically? We can control our pain with a painkiller and then continue. In this, our behaviour is clearly different from that of other animals. An animal that is in pain will still do what is necessary to survive, but otherwise, it will respond to what it feels. In the case of pain, an animal will reduce or even stop its activities. But humans? Based on their intellect and social context (deadlines, caring for the family), they will continue their activities wherever possible. Supported perhaps by some form of pain suppression. Through pain, the nervous system communicates that, given the circumstances, the body is overloaded. Regardless of whether there is physical damage, the nervous system notices that the body has not sufficiently adjusted its level of activity to the situation. The nervous system concludes that the given pain signal is not being anticipated properly. Apparently, the signal is not being detected sufficiently. The solution of the nervous system is to allow the pain signal to come through more intensely. The mechanism by which the nervous system does this? Sensitisation.
The effect is that pain worsens. Not because of (imminent) tissue damage but because behaviour is not adequately adjusted. This may explain why patients with chronic pain in the Spine & Joint

Centre experience a decrease in pain in such a short time as soon as they start taking their rest periods. Taking rest is apparently a behavioural change that the nervous system considers necessary. Finally, the body does what has been suggested for so long (by the nervous system): it relieves the pressure in the body. As a result, sensitisation decreases and even faster than expected. Apparently, it is not so much a structural change in the brain but an alarm system that is constantly on. Not because it was out of order but because the underlying problem, the necessary behavioural change, did not come. Until the behaviour actually changed.

The essence of pain
In essence, pain is a warning mechanism in our body. Under certain exceptional circumstances, it can get out of control and cause pain for no 'reason'. These situations are very, very rare. It can occur with tumours, after an amputation or after some kinds of surgery, or after a viral infection of the nerve pathways. This can happen occasionally. It has nothing to do with the many people who experience persistent back, pelvic or neck pain. Or other pains somewhere in their body.
What we propose is to go back to the essence of pain. The premise that, in the vast majority of cases, pain is simply trying to warn us. And we humans are no longer so good at listening to what the body wants to tell us. If we want our pain to decrease, we should not suppress it (too quickly) or cut it away. It might be much more effective to

respect pain and its function. Perhaps we should adjust our priorities and adapt our actions, just like animals do.

9. Pain as Pain Is Intended

'You have enemies? Good. That means you've stood up for something, sometime in your life.'
-Winston Churchill

JP: 'This understanding of pain in animals puts the way we deal with pain in a different perspective.'
Vince: 'Yes, right? Although we can reduce pain medically and technically, it could be that some interventions are counterproductive.'
JP: 'We are also stubborn people who just want to continue with our daily activities, which we consider important. Of course, that is not convenient either.'
Vince: 'On the other hand, there are certainly situations in which it is very convenient that pain can be suppressed or stopped altogether.'
JP: 'So it is difficult to give one answer to the question of how to deal with pain. It is complex and nuanced. Would it be an idea to put a number of things into perspective in this chapter?'
Vince: 'Certainly, but keep in mind: it is not a question of right or wrong; there are simply different ways of looking at it. If we allow ourselves to add the perspective that we describe here, it may open up new possibilities for pain treatment.'

Monkey Business

Journey
In this book, we have taken you on a journey of discovery. In doing so, we have sought answers to the question of where our pain system comes from. We have discovered that the origin of our pain system is incredibly old and fundamental. A form of protection had to be organised from the very beginning in the first single-celled organisms. From an evolutionary perspective, this makes sense. Organisms that end up in a dangerous or potentially deadly situation have less chance of survival and will probably not last millions of years.

Different pain systems
Although all animals seem to be equipped with warning systems (a pain system), these systems can vary between species. However, in mammals, these warning systems – both neurological and hormonal – appear to be very similar. This has led to the question of whether, apart from humans, mammals and even non-mammals can experience pain. This question is complex because the experience of 'pain' is the subjective interpretation of the perception of internal stimuli (including nociceptive stimuli). The simplistic idea that animals cannot experience pain because they do not express it is now really outdated. There is a growing body of animal research showing that animals exhibit specific behaviours of a type that indicates animals do indeed experience something we would call pain. The fact that they cannot express pain with words

cannot be used as an argument that they do not feel pain. Furthermore, when we talk to each other about our pain, we can never fully understand what the other person is feeling or experiencing. What we can do is imagine how it would feel for us if we were in a similar situation. We then assume that this feeling is probably what the other person is experiencing.

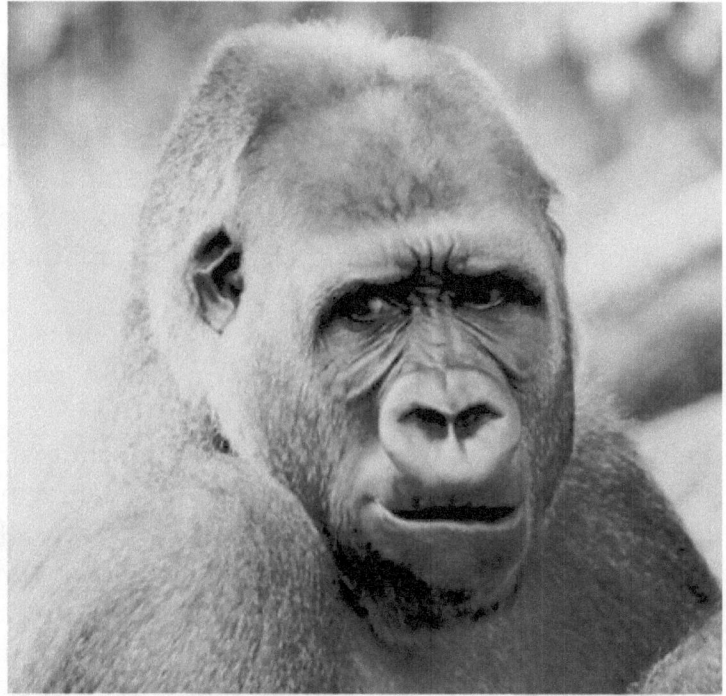

Western lowland gorilla (Gorilla gorilla gorilla). To what extent are we able to understand the facial expressions of other animals? Photo: Jan-Paul

This is very similar to the situation with animals, we can only rely on the behaviour and/or facial expression of the animal (as we should do with humans). The problem is that we are simply not adept at understanding the behaviour and facial expressions of animals. For example, to determine whether an animal is in pain, we mainly look for changes in their metabolism. Think of factors such as food intake, digestion, breathing patterns, body temperature or blood pressure. Disruptions of these parameters can indicate that an animal is in pain. This way of measuring helps and supports our understanding of pain in animals. But it remains difficult. Analogous to the question posed in the book by the famous behavioural scientist Frans de Waal, *Are we smart enough to understand how smart animals are?* We can ask something similar about empathising with animals. Are we empathetic enough to feel what animals feel?

Pain: Protection, behaviour control or learning system?
Pain is supposed to be a protective mechanism. Usually, we have already responded to a damaging or threatening situation before we actually experience the pain. It seems very likely that experiencing pain is not a primary but rather a secondary part of our protective mechanism. Experiencing pain makes us pay attention to the painful area; we avoid further potentially harmful contact and pay attention to the sore spot. Dogs and cats do this by licking the injured area, people by putting a plaster, bandage or ointment on it or by holding or rubbing the painful body part. Pain helps

us to learn; 'Oops, that was not a smart move to put my hand under the hot tap. I had better avoid that next time.' Experiencing pain therefore seems to be strongly linked to learning processes and complex behavioural adjustments.

Pain behaviour
Despite their similar pain systems, mammals can display very different pain behaviours. This behaviour depends on the type of animal. A predator in pain behaves differently than a prey animal in pain. The living environment also plays an important role. The female macaques giving birth are probably all in pain. The extent to which they express their pain depends largely on their living environment and in particular their perceived degree of safety. The safer they are, the more they express the pain they experience.
The pain behaviour of macaques already resembles the way humans deal with pain. However, the differences between people are even greater. Although much knowledge is still lacking, it is becoming increasingly clear that cultural evolution and the phenomenon of intersubjective truth play an enormously important role in the way we deal with pain.

Cultural evolution
Cultural evolution has taken a huge leap forward in humans, especially through the intensive use of language. Through language, we give meaning to our observations. Unfortunately, being able to put

experiences into words can work in different – positive and negative – directions. When we discover a lump somewhere in our body, we can interpret it as a 'fatty lump', but equally well as a 'tumour'. Giving such a specific meaning to a finding is not without a price. Emotions, or evaluative feelings, are always connected to these words. A fatty lump is not harmful and will not upset us very much, but the image of a potentially fatal tumour will strongly activate our stress system. In such a case, in line with the stress system, our pain system will also be stimulated and become more sensitive to sensations around the lump (sensitisation). The area around the lump becomes more sensitive, and this increased sensitivity can again confirm the idea that there is very likely something seriously wrong.

Neurogenic dysregulation as a misconception
This brings us to the supposed dysregulation of our pain system. It is strange, to say the least, that a system that has evolved in humans over millions of years can suddenly go astray and malfunction. Such an event is highly unlikely. Sensitisation is a normal physiological mechanism necessary for the pain system. We need to stop blaming our nervous system. It is not (dysregulation of) our nervous system that causes persistent pain but our own persistent behaviour. This is good news for people with persistent pain. In many cases, it is possible to reduce pain. The idea that sensitisation causes permanent, lasting pain is outdated and no longer valid. Sensitisation is just one part of how our

nervous system works. It contributes to a heightened experience of pain when necessary but has the ability to normalise when circumstances permit.

Thinking (cognitions) and feelings
Our cognitions, the way we think about our complaints, influences our pain experience. In other words, the image we create about what we feel has a great influence on how we feel about it. Because of this relationship, it is only logical that science focuses on the psychological possibilities of pain treatments. Psychological treatments are sometimes successful, but not always. Sometimes patients continue to have pain. The pain does not decrease and might even get worse. Why is the psychological approach not always successful? What are we missing? Let's go back to animals.
In animal rehabilitation, it is essential that the animal starts to show a certain behaviour. Behaviour that helps their body recover. Of course, it is not possible to verbally convey the intention of an exercise to the animal. After all, animals do not have the ability to understand human language. Although there are many owners who claim that their pet understands them perfectly. How rehabilitation works in animals is by physically inviting or stimulating them to show the desired behaviour.

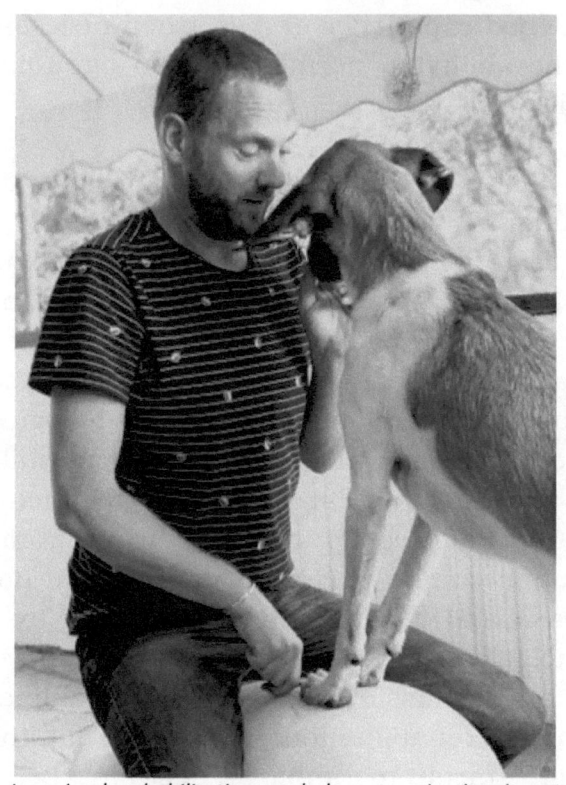

In animal rehabilitation, verbal communication is not necessary. The response of an animal (in this case, Gaia) is directly related to what is experienced. Photo: Jeffrey Singh

Once they experience a positive response to their modified behaviour, it is amazing how quickly their body adapts and incorporates the new behaviour. The main point here is that animals do not think. Their behaviour is based on more or less direct reactions to their experiences. The newly learned behaviour, if experienced positively, will normalise and become part of their normal movement behaviour. Cognitive pondering, as people tend to do, can be an obstacle in the experience process: 'Am I doing the exercise right?' 'Should I exercise harder?' 'Can this harm my body?' 'Does the therapist see that I am really trying?'

This is the big difference between psychological pain treatments and animal rehabilitation. The paths that are taken are exactly opposite. Animals adapt the 'image' of what they can do based on their experience. Whereas in the psychological approach, humans must first be cognitively 'convinced' before a positive experience can be gained. The simple phrase, 'Just try it, it can't do any harm...' can trigger a cascade of thoughts, considerations and mental obstacles in a patient with pain complaints. An animal suffers much less from this.

It is precisely our intensive use of language that makes it necessary to first cognitively convince people that a certain movement is possible, and then to have them perform the movement. From a biological perspective, it is much more effective to change the image directly from the physical experience. In our modern Western world, this is called 'being in the here and now', but it actually comes down to bypassing our constantly thinking brains.

It does not mean that animals do not consider their options. A dog that is careful with waves will not jump into the sea just because cheese is handed out. They are still considering their options, and somehow, they decide which behaviour is desirable at that moment.

Monkey Business

Practical applicability
Some time ago, at the end of a course we held on pain in animals and people, we received this feedback: 'A beautiful perspective, but what can we, as practitioners do with this in our daily practice?' A completely justified and logical question. Unfortunately, it is also a question that is not so easy to answer. There is simply no fixed recipe for optimal treatment, despite the wish of many practitioners: 'If the patient has this, prepare this recipe or perform this treatment.' Unfortunately, it does not work that way.

In this book, we look critically at a number of aspects of pain from the perspective of animals and discuss various consequences that emerge in relation to human pain perception. How and when these consequences influence a treatment is up to the practitioner, the patient and the situation. However, we will not send the reader into practice empty-handed. In the following paragraphs, we discuss some of the practical consequences. Some will be new for you or even unconventional. Some may already be known or be obvious. However, we feel it is important to mention them again because they are essential aspects of how we view pain.

Accept someone's pain
Pain is an individual, personal experience. In humans, the degree to which someone says they are in pain does not necessarily correspond to the behaviour we observe. Unconsciously, or sometimes consciously, we compare verbal and

nonverbal behaviour, and we expect a certain degree of congruence between them. The absence of congruence seems strange or even suspicious to us. Of course, we know that on the one hand, there are those who persevere through their pain and do not seem to feel it, and on the other hand, there are the wimps who squeak at the slightest injury. There is a margin in how 'true' we find someone's pain, depending on our image of the person in question. Interpreting someone's pain becomes more complicated if that person also comes from a different culture. The display of the degree of pain and the way in which it is expressed varies greatly between cultures. Think back to the story of the macaque monkeys. Culture and environment have a great influence on pain behaviour. This brings us back to the fundamental problem of not knowing how another individual, animal or human, experiences their pain. An important starting point is therefore to accept it as a given when someone indicates that they are in pain. Acceptance of the indication of pain does not mean that something should be done about it.

Pain behaviour can have different functions in humans and animals. The task of a practitioner is to determine the 'function' of the pain in the specific situation. Is it mainly protective? Or does the pain behaviour also have a social function: 'Please help me because I am in a very bad way.' A good example is the difference in the changes in pain between European people and people from the Middle East. During pain treatment at the Spine & Joint Centre, it is customary to check at certain points during the process whether the patient's pain has changed. Europeans normally experience a slow decrease in pain during the course of the treatment. To our initial surprise, and especially frustration, this decrease in pain is much less in people from the Middle East. They indicate that they experience pain for longer. Their pain level remains virtually unchanged during the treatment. This is the case even as their physical functioning visibly improves. From their perspective, they are patients, and within their cultural context, pain is part of that experience. Only when the treatment is finished do the pain scores decrease. This is, of course, a generalization with large individual differences. In general, however, these cultural differences are clearly observable.

Message from the patient
Pain should not persist under normal circumstances. In pathological cases, such as those involving amputations or post-operative situations, pain may persist, which can be considered a natural, physiological response of the nervous system to a pathological and/or structurally altered situation. In all other situations, one should always ask why pain persists. Pain is primarily a signal that something is wrong in the body. As already indicated, pain behaviour can serve many other functions besides physical complaints. To make matters even more complicated, there may be an underlying physical problem that causes someone

to experience pain, but they adjust their pain behaviour based on the social context. This can have very different effects. For example, some people may tolerate their pain and continue as if nothing is wrong, while others may exaggerate their pain behaviour to send a social signal: 'help me' or 'comfort me'. These different forms of pain behaviour also have physical consequences. The first category of individuals may ignore the underlying physical problems which causes the body to become overloaded and the physical problems to increase over time. In the second category, individuals avoid using their bodies, leading to avoidance behaviour and physical deconditioning. These are just a few examples of the many possible nuances of pain behaviour that exist in practice. The trick is to map the behaviour pattern of the patient with pain. However, behaviour patterns are not static, which adds an extra layer of complexity. People can change their behaviour over time, depending on their emotional state or their changed physical or social situation.

Pain relief or finding a solution
What could be more satisfying for a practitioner than to relieve someone's pain? This is precisely what many treatments focus on: the immediate removal of pain. To reduce pain, practitioners have a variety of methods at their disposal, including massage, deep transverse friction, manipulation, hot packs, TENS, fascia techniques or more exotic techniques such as dry needling and cupping.

These techniques can indeed provide some relief, but unfortunately, it often only lasts for a short time. Only in cases where pain remains absent is the treatment really effective. But what happens if the pain returns after a few hours or days?
We are making a crucial mistake here. Removing pain (a symptom) makes the underlying problem more difficult to understand. The practitioner is faced with a fundamental choice here: relieve the pain or – if possible – solve the underlying problem. This choice leads to very different treatment strategies. For a good practitioner, the choice will not be difficult.

Pain medication can enhance pain
Nowadays, there are various pain medications available – some by prescription at pharmacies and many others on drugstore shelves. Access to such medications allows us to suppress our pain for a while, which is useful when we want to work or go to a party. However, there are several disadvantages to using painkillers. For example, the effectiveness of some medications is questionable, while other, stronger medications can have serious side effects. One aspect of painkillers that is less well-known is that they can make your pain worse in the long run. Only when the danger has been averted can the pain return to perform its protective function. A similar process occurs with the use of painkillers, the medication allows us to continue our activities, but such behaviour carries risks for the body. Just like the danger, when the effect of the medication

wears off, the pain can be experienced more intensely. Your nervous system has noticed that there has been no or insufficient response to the previous pain signals. This mechanism of pain medication in combination with unchanged behaviour can worsen the pain in the long term.

Thoughts on the run
Did you ever imagine a monster under your bed as a child? The thought of the monster becomes increasingly intense until you are sitting in your bed crying with fear. In this way, we can imagine all sorts of things about the possible causes of the pain we experience. Such images are not innocent. They always have an emotional component. Just like with the crying toddler, images and thoughts can trigger an emotional rollercoaster. This also applies to our pain mechanisms. This phenomenon emphasises the importance of transferring adequate information to patients. An area in which shortcomings are often apparent. By having exercises performed without explaining the purpose of the exercise and what the patient can expect, you can completely miss the mark.

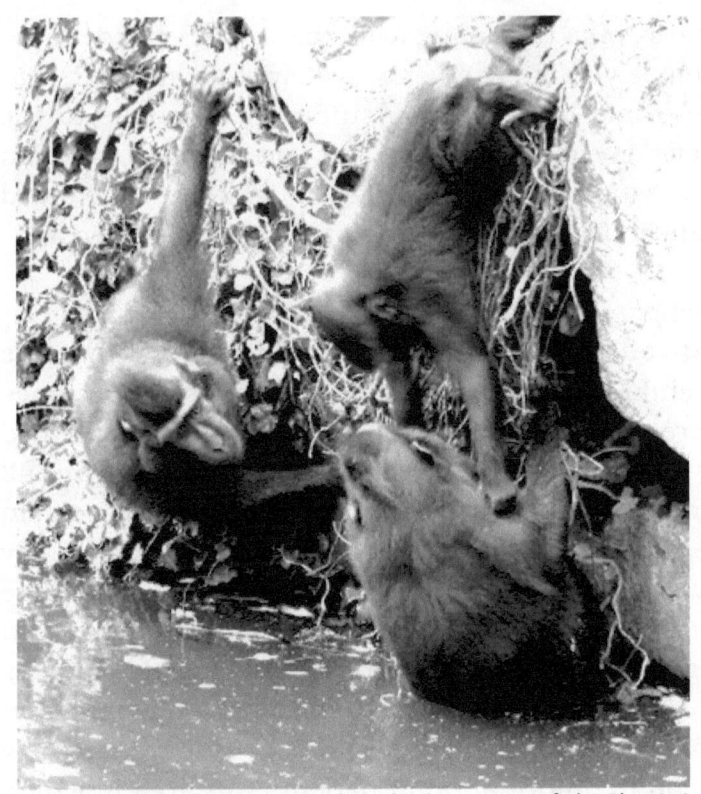

Crested macaques (Macaca Nigra) involved in a serious fight. The victim has fled into the water. Photo: Jan-Paul

It works much better if you, as a practitioner, indicate in advance what the purpose of the exercise is and when more or less pain might be experienced. If you do this, the potentially negative effect of 'more pain' will be converted into a positive experience: after all, this is what could be expected. According to the expert (the practitioner), this is logical and normal, and I (the patient) can trust this. Such thought patterns have a dampening effect on the nervous system. This is also what is described in the book *Explain Pain* by David Butler and Lorimer Mosely. Although moderating images and thoughts can help, this is certainly not the whole story.

The illusion of a difference between acute and chronic pain
Nowadays, it is common to distinguish between acute and chronic pain. This peculiar distinction is generally accepted and seems beyond discussion. The distinction between 'acute' and 'chronic' is mainly based on time. The applicable period varies from six weeks to three or even six months. After this period of time, damaged tissue is expected to have healed. Pain after this period can no longer be associated with tissue damage. Tissues have had ample time to recover. Apart from exceptions such as those resulting from a vegetative disorder that slows down recovery processes, it is clear that after this period, damaged tissue can no longer be the cause of pain. This poses a problem for doctors and scientists. If tissue damage cannot explain pain, what can? Even though one could imagine other causes, science came up with sensitization: the dysregulation of the nervous system. And with sensitisation came psychology. After all, it are our thoughts and fears that maintain the process of sensitisation.
Let us examine this strange train of thought again. First of all, it is illogical to assume that tissue will 'by definition' repair itself within a certain period of time. Under normal circumstances, biological tissue will indeed repair itself within a certain

period of time. But the circumstances are not taken into account. Is it not possible that someone might do something or perform a certain activity that repeatedly forces or damages the tissue? In this case recovery will take much longer or perhaps not at all. Think of a marathon runner with an Achilles tendon injury. If this athlete wants to continue to run his weekly kilometres, he will probably not recover. Even significantly reducing the kilometres that he runs will not be enough. Only with sufficient rest can the body recover.

So, a problem such as this does not persist because there is some obscure chronic aspect to it; it persists simply because the body is repeatedly damaged or overloaded.

The second point is the idea that it takes weeks or even months for sensitisation to occur. As already described, sensitisation occurs almost immediately when necessary. It is part of our normal physiological response to injury. Sensitisation is an essential mechanism for the nervous system to draw attention to damaged body parts or tissues. Sensitisation certainly does not only begin at the transition from acute to chronic.

It is therefore a strange idea to assume that biological systems will suddenly behave very differently based on time. Biological systems are mainly dependent on circumstances and not so much on time. If we want to understand physical recovery processes and abnormal healing, it is better to look at the circumstances and how the body reacts, instead of just relying on the time that has passed.

So, it is possible that within a very short period of time (hours to days), depending on the circumstances, a physical problem with a 'chronic' character could arise. On the other hand, one can suffer from a physical problem for months that still has an 'acute' character.

We believe that it is time to let go of the artificial distinction between acute and chronic as it is currently maintained and to instead focus on the recovery process itself.

> **The limbic system** is evolutionarily one of the oldest parts of the brain. It is part of the cerebrum and is involved in emotion, motivation, pleasure and pain responses, and emotional memory. Emotion mainly comes from the limbic system and it has a lot to do with the formation of memories.

The importance of positive emotional responses

Humans have high-level cognitive abilities and are able to gather and share knowledge. Our cognitive abilities not only help us survive but also enable us to create a beneficial world around us. As we have described in the previous paragraphs, it is very useful to cognitively understand what happens in our body when we experience pain. What is less noticeable is that there is a much more important neurological system running in the background that has more control than we are aware of; the limbic (emotion) system.

Monkey Business

Everything we perceive is unconsciously linked to a cognitive-emotional charge. This emotional charge largely determines how our body reacts. Here, we are not only talking about directly visible behaviour but also about less directly visible physiological responses such as heart rate, breathing, blood pressure and vasoconstriction or dilation. For many of these observations, the practical impact on our physical system is minimal (e.g., do I pick up my bag or not?). Such a simple consideration becomes more complicated when you have back problems. For example, you could have the underlying thought (cognition) that the action of 'picking up a bag' can damage your back. Your emotional system, activated by this image, can make you hesitate to pick up your bag. Then you remember that your phone is in the bag and that you really need it. There is also an emotional component to this thought: 'I really need my phone.' Your brain will weigh the risk of pain against the necessity of having your phone in your hands. When your need to have your phone prevails, you pick up the bag. If this action is painful, it can make you even more reluctant the next time you have to bend down. Then a (smart) therapist notices the tense behaviour of the patient and gives him the following instruction: 'Relax your back and let it move more freely. Try to bend forward with less tension.' The patient will weigh this instruction cognitively-emotionally and ask themselves the ultimate question: 'Am I going to do this or not?' There is trust in the therapist (based on previous positive experiences) and at the same time, there is the fear of pain. Let us say for the moment that the patient chooses to follow the advice and is able to move in a more relaxed way. Bending forward succeeds and the patient feels that the movement is much less painful. This experience makes connections in different brain areas. The first is a cognitive link: I am able to bend forward with less pain if I do it this way. Second, this experience affects the emotional system: after the positive experience, the emotional state becomes more relaxed, and the aroused state decreases. This experience also has an effect on other emotional levels. For example, trust in the therapist is strengthened: the therapist was right, I can trust him/her. With literally everything we think or imagine, there is always an emotional connection in the background. Who hasn't had the experience of going somewhere and looking forward to it but at the same time, having an unconscious idea that something doesn't feel right? In that scenario, your limbic system is activated because it hates the event you're attending, while at the same time, your cognitive brain keeps telling you that you should like it. 'Go with your gut' basically means don't overthink it, but pay more attention to what your limbic system is telling you.

Motivation comes from experience
Motivation is not a character trait; it is the dynamic result of a complex of cognitive-emotional factors. Motivation can change from moment to moment, depending on the circumstances. Take a child who

sees candy on the table. Some motivators, such as the thought of the sweet taste of the candy, will stimulate the child to take the candy. Other motivators will have an inhibiting effect. For example, the thought that someone might get angry. Many more subtle emotions play a role than we can describe here, such as past experiences and the degree of desire for the candy. And then, when the child has just decided to take the candy and is on his way to the table, the sound of footsteps on the stairs can be enough for the child to leave the candy there. A similar dynamic response occurs around pain. Pain is a strong motivator and therefore a strong emotional stimulus, aimed at preventing possible harmful actions. The more a patient experiences movements or activities that can be performed without pain, the less reluctant he will be to perform those actions. If the patient experiences (increasing) pain during an activity, it will become increasingly difficult to continue performing the actions and the patient will eventually give up. This is an important problem with Graded Exposure and Graded Activity; patients are initially willing to comply with the therapist's instructions. If negative feedback (i.e. pain) persists for too long or even increases, the patient will quickly become reluctant to perform the exercises.

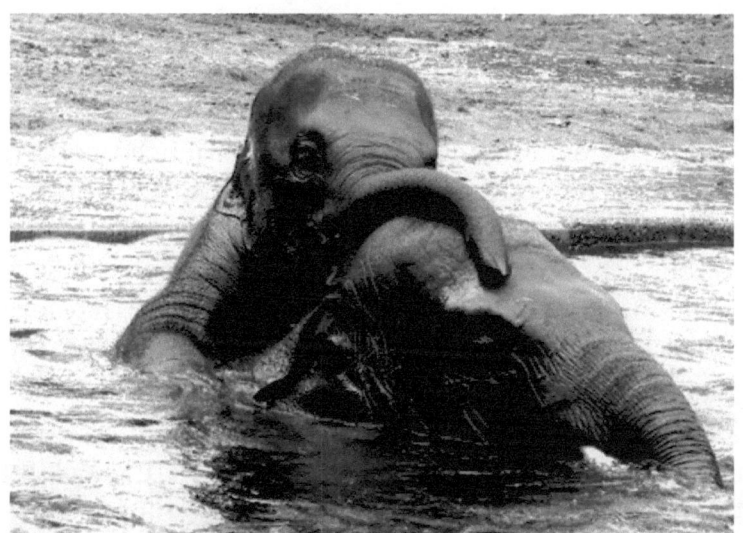

Asian elephants (Elephas maximus) play in the water, a seemingly useless activity. Apparently, they find it very enjoyable and can keep it up for a long time. Photo: Jan-Paul

The problem with Graded Exposure and Graded Activity

Treatments such as Graded Exposure and Graded Activity come from the psychological domain. The premise is that in people with persistent pain, there is nothing wrong with the body. Therefore, it is assumed that the body can be loaded as long as the load level is below a 'no-failure' level – the level over which the body cannot be expected to be forced or overloaded in any way. In Graded Exposure, patients are increasingly exposed to movements and activities that they believe will damage their body or cause them pain. In Graded Activity, the load level is increased, regardless of the pain experienced – after all, there is nothing wrong with the body! The ultimate goal of these treatments is for patients to be able to resume their daily activities as much as possible, regardless of the pain they experience. The pain experienced is seen as a poor perception of the nervous system, and the patient must learn to ignore the abnormal signals. Such psychologically-based treatments are sometimes successful, but just as often, they are not. We have seen above that pain is one of the strongest motivators to stop activities (that cause pain). We must therefore realise that these behavioural treatments try to get patients moving via a motivationally-weak cognitive route. It is actually a miracle that patients actually improve via these programs. However, these results can be explained – partly. All these programs start with low load levels. Levels at which the body can apply normal motor strategies. It is conceivable that some patients, as a coincidental result, start to use their bodies in better balance. This can lead to a recovery of function and consequently, a decrease in pain. It is a pity that this effect from these programs occurs essentially by chance. It would be more effective if this balancing of the body were the main goal of the therapy.

The malleable world and the nature of pain
In our Western world, we have a pleasant life. We live in a safe environment, in homes with all kinds of conveniences and comforts. We have enough to eat. If we have a problem, there are all kinds of ways to solve our problem. We can insure ourselves

against many possible inconveniences, such as damage, loss or theft of our property. We can even insure ourselves against illness through our health insurance. All this gives us the feeling that our lives and our health are malleable and controllable. Pain is viewed in the same way. We believe that pain should be malleable or at least manageable. By thinking this way, incredibly, we ignore the nature of pain. Pain is our old, faithful warning system. Over the centuries, pain has learned all kinds of ways to continue to be heard. Pain will not be silent as long as the organism to which it belongs (you) has not adequately adjusted its behaviour. If the pain is blocked by medication or injection, it will look for ways to continue to warn you. Because that is the purpose of pain.

This nature of pain is at odds with our desire to control our body and our feelings. With all good intentions, pain is very persistent and annoying in its goal which is to warn you. The fact that you are not waiting for that warning: pain does not care. You need to be protected.

It may be that the more we try to suppress pain, the harder and more fiercely it will keep coming back. The solution here is to change your attitude towards pain. Stop pushing it away and investigate what the pain is trying to tell you.

Of course, this strategy will not work for all forms of persistent pain. However, even in the case of pain after amputation or with tumours, stopping the struggle and trying to adopt different behaviour often yields very positive results. This is not about 'resignation' or 'acceptance' in the sense of 'resigning yourself to it'. These are often passive strategies. What is meant here is consciously looking for other ways to deal with the pain.

An integrated approach for the treatment of pain
With all that we have described here about pain, it seems unwise to leave the treatment of pain to a single discipline. As science shows, pain is multifactorial, with the body, mind and environment each playing their part. Psychologists (with all due respect) mainly understand and deal with the way we think. Psychology is less about how we feel and certainly not about the way we move. Physiotherapists understand more about the body but less about the mind.

So, instead of assigning pain treatments to a single discipline, it seems wiser to divide tasks and work together for optimal results. How we think about things and how we can influence those thoughts is an important factor in effectively combating pain. This learning process is similar in both animals and humans. We learn and adapt our behaviour based on our experiences. The only difference is that humans also use words and assign a subjective charge to those words. The ability to use words is powerful, but unfortunately, it works in two ways: it can be both helpful and harmful. That is why it is wise for doctors, specialists and psychologists to work together with therapists who understand the body. Actually, a behavioural scientist or perhaps even a sales expert would also be part of it.

Someone who understands how motivation works, not motivation from words but, as with animals, motivation based on perception and (physical) awareness.

So, back to our roots
Fundamentally, our bodies differ very little from those of other mammals. The same applies to our cognitive skills. Our level of thinking may also be less far removed from other animals than we sometimes think. Our use of language and words, in which we distinguish ourselves from other animals, does make a big difference. Linguistic thinking enables us to conduct scientific studies and thus develop our knowledge of pain and pain systems. At the same time, thinking with language creates a sneaky pitfall. We have created the illusion for ourselves that we can solve all problems with our language skills. But if you are hungry, you may be able to 'think' that hunger away for a while. Ultimately, you cannot solve your hunger by thinking and it is not the case that we can solve the hunger in the world by cutting nerve pathways. If you are hungry, the message is you have to eat something. Or better, trust your hunger because it is telling you what you want.

It is no different with pain. We can think and assume all sorts of things about our pain, but it all starts with feeling and experiencing what the pain wants to tell us. We can't get around that. We have to go back to our roots. Back to the human animal that we are, who can still feel and experience in addition to thinking. It could well be that experiencing pain and our 'primitive' basic reaction to it can do a lot for us. We don't have to let go of our acquired knowledge and insights. We have to learn to keep using them in combination with feeling and experiencing what pain actually wants to tell us. We then to act accordingly. Just like all other animals, we are and will remain simple creatures. But very special creatures, that's for sure.

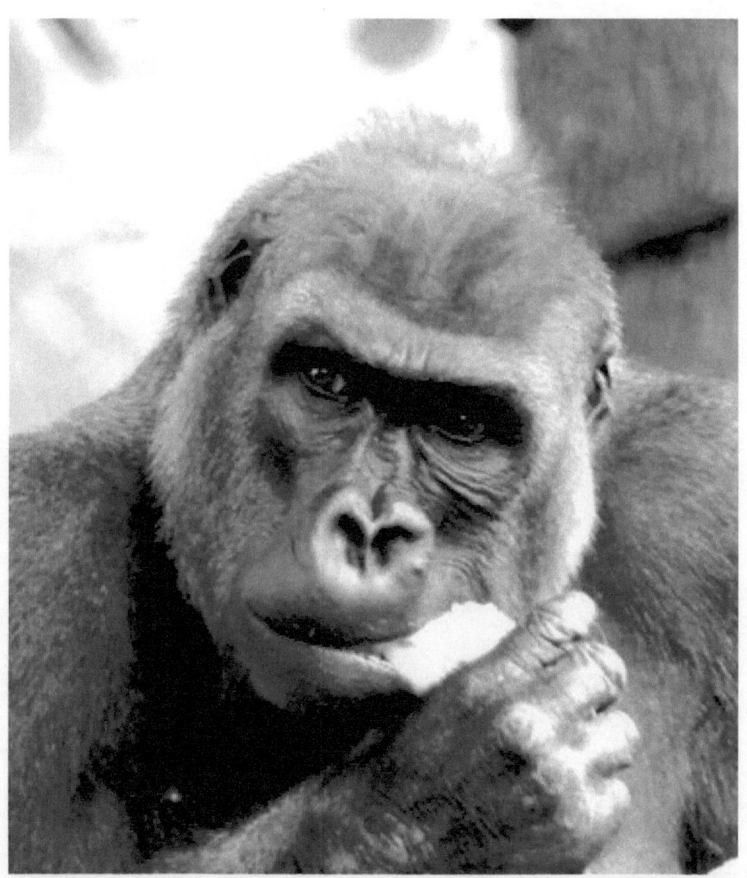

Western lowland gorilla (Gorilla gorilla gorilla). We are so full of our cognitive abilities. Will species like this gorilla eventually gain the ability to use language, just like us? And will this be an unqualified advantage for them? Photo: Jan-Paul

10. Epilogue

'Why this book had to be written'

Both Vincent and Jan-Paul have had experiences with people who had persistent pain. Sometimes in a similar way, sometimes very differently. Below, they give you their own motivations as to why they found writing this book important.

'Oook!'
-The librarian, Discworld, Terry Pratchett

Jan-Paul:
My first real encounter with people with persistent pain was in 1996. The Spine & Joint Centre was founded to treat patients with pelvic girdle pain after pregnancy. Years earlier, a research group from Erasmus University developed a model that helped us understand how pelvic complaints can arise. I will never forget how difficult it was to convince women with pelvic pain not to overload themselves. In order to reduce overload and irritation in their pelvic joints and to enable recovery, these women had to limit their activities and rest more often. And if there is one thing that women who have just become mothers do not want, it is to rest. Their goal is to take care of their child

and family. The main purpose for which they were put on this earth and nothing will stop them. No pelvic pain or stupid therapist could convince them otherwise.

At that moment, we realised that simply offering exercises to someone with chronic pain was not going to work. We had to be psychologically smarter. We needed to understand what drives and motivates patients. An effective treatment for this patient group includes not only physical but also psychological and behavioural aspects. For example, we started our integrated rehabilitation treatment to address back, pelvic and neck complaints.

This specific rehabilitation program falls under the category of 'chronic pain' as defined by the government and health insurance companies. Initially this was not a problem. These women and men had pain and it was chronic, so they met the criteria.

Over the years, the images of chronic pain have developed further. This development also led to a polarization of perspectives. The biopsychosocial model gained popularity. In daily practice, this led to a shift towards a more psychological treatment approach, in which physical aspects were increasingly disregarded.

What we call interdisciplinary treatment is often no more than a number of serial sessions with different disciplines. What is not sufficiently understood is that physical exercises provide incredible emotional feedback. If performed well, this can help change the way patients think. Unfortunately, in current treatments, each discipline only addresses its own safe area of expertise. We need to start realising that this doesn't work and never will. As Descartes suggested, we humans don't have separate bodies and minds. We are bodies, with our own psyches, unique social problems and unique ergonomic challenges. We are creatures trying to live, survive and reproduce in our environment. Just like any other creature.

I hate to admit it, but I myself have a chronic pain problem. For years, I have suffered from inflammation in my left foot, particularly in the big toe. At first, I thought I had injured my toe. The pain and inflammation subsided and I thought that was the end of it. However the inflammation and pain returned. The frequency and duration of the pain increased over time. I tried everything: bandages, tape, different shoes, painkillers, anti-inflammatories, exercise and rest. Nothing solved the problem permanently. I spent sleepless nights trying to get my foot into a position where the pain would be bearable. I was unaware that I had had this 'incidental' condition for over ten years. It was so insidious and creeping that I never realised how bad it had become. Then there is the story about a patient who came to us for treatment and said to our secretary: 'I wonder if I am the right patient here because that man is in much worse shape.' That man was me, hobbling up the stairs to get to work. Over time, my left leg had shrunk to half the size of my right. I literally fell off my bike once. When I fell six meters down a flight of stairs because I lost control, the limit had been reached. This was not good. In desperation, I went to a rheumatologist. The specialist listened to my story for five minutes before concluding that I probably had gout. I expected a future of endless blood tests and imaging techniques. But no, during the consultation, she carefully inserted a needle into my painful toe joint, extracted some synovial fluid and placed it under a microscope. Almost immediately, she said: 'Look, there's one there, and there's another one.' I was allowed to take a look through the microscope. In the synovial fluid, the blue-green glow of the urea crystals was easy to see. This was gout! I was given medication that same day, and from that moment on, I never experienced that terrible pain again. A true miracle. Every now and then, I experience a certain feeling around my toe. Even though I haven't had an attack in years, my mind still goes; 'Oh my god, here we go again.' Even though I haven't had pain in my toe in years, my brain still seems to be very focused on what could happen to my toe. Once a patient with pain, always a patient with pain.

In the many conversations I had with Vincent about this subject, we agreed on many points. Although it often took a while before we figured it out. Our discussions are often intense but always constructive. The subject of pain is not easy or clear-cut. There is so much that is simply not yet known. But it is time to look at the pain problem differently. In doing so, we want to look as much as possible at what is really there. The examples of animals that Vincent brought to this book are wonderful material for this. Hopefully, this book will help you to look at people differently. Not as a 'person with pain' but as an animal trying to survive. With that, our view of pain and how to deal with it can fundamentally change.

'In natural science the principles of truth ought to be confirmed by observation.'
-Carl Linnaeus

Vincent:
I believe that humans are the strangest of all animals. By that, I mean that our behaviour as a species deviates greatly from our natural behaviour. And I also agree with Frans de Waal that human dominance on earth is overestimated. We are inclined to want to prove that we are different from other mammals. But are we really that different? Especially when it comes to pain, we can learn more from our similarities than from our differences. By focusing on the differences, we mainly emphasise the uniqueness and special nature of humans. Focusing on the similarities, on the other hand, makes us humble and grounded within biology. This tacking between differences and similarities among species intensified the conversations we had while writing this book.

With the current, predominantly psychological approach to chronic pain, it seems wise to also listen to what the biological or evolutionary approach tells us. Before we reduce pain to a mental disorder, we should ask ourselves whether that is justified. When I started working with animals, which have a biologically and neurologically pain system similar to humans, I discovered how language basically plays no role at all. The low self-esteem of a cat, the beliefs of a horse and the high workload of a dog are non-existent. What they do, their behaviour, is very relevant and the most valuable and reliable source of information. The latest hype in the human pain industry is about placebos and nocebos. The dogs I treat at the local shelter for chronic pain, the ones with anatomical abnormalities, are they eagerly awaiting the results of meta-analyses on placebo effects and other convictions that contribute to chronic pain in humans??

My relationship with Jan-Paul goes back a long way. In 1999, he was my internship supervisor at the Spine & Joint Centre, but we quickly became good friends. One of the nicest things about our friendship is that we regularly try to prove each other wrong. A normal and common behaviour in young hominidea. Our conversations are challenging and because we are both competitive and like to base things on facts ('evidence'), we help each other further in life. We help each other further in our understanding of pain. Pain in both human and non-human animals. Hence this book. Thank you, Jeep, for all your wise lessons, opportunities, help and for your friendship. I sincerely hope that we continue to challenge ourselves and each other in the coming years, with lots of wine, food and laughter.

11. Literature

This book is not written in a scientific style. For the sake of readability, it was decided not to interrupt the text with literature references, as is customary in scientific texts. However, the content of the book is thoroughly supported with scientific literature where possible. As shown in the book, it is not about science itself, it is about the way in which we interpret and use scientific findings.

For the interested reader who wants to delve deeper into the scientific side of this book, we have added the most important references to articles, books and other sources.

Apkarian AV, Bushnell MC, Treede RD, Zubieta JK. (2005) Human brain mechanisms of pain perception and regulation in health and disease. *Eur J Pain.* Aug; 9(4):463-84.

Arias-Carrión O, Pöppel E. (2007) Dopamine, learning, and reward-seeking behaviour. *Acta Neurobiol Exp (Wars).* 67(4):481-8.

Bajcar EA, Bąbel P. (2024) Social learning of placebo effects in pain: a critical review of the literature and a proposed revised model. *J Pain.* May; 31:104585.

Bockstahler B et al. (2019) *Essential Facts of Physical Medicine, Rehabilitation and Sports*

Medicine in Companion Animals. VBS GmbH, Babenhausen, Germany.

Bonavita V, De Simone R. (2011) Pain as an evolutionary necessity. *Neurol Sci.* May; 32 Suppl 1:S61-6.

Braithwaite V. (2010) *Do Fish Feel Pain?* Oxford University Press, Incorporated.

Bregman R. (2019) De meeste mensen deugen: een nieuwe geschiedenis van de mens (Dutch Edition) (01 editie) [Eng: Humankind: A Hopeful History]. De Correspondent BV.

Bristol Adam S et al. (2004) Neural circuit of tail-elicited siphon withdrawal in Aplysia. II. Role of gated inhibition in differential lateralization of sensitization and dishabituation. *J Neurophysiol.* 91: 678– 692.

Browe BM, Vice EN, Park TJ. (2020) The naked mole rats: Blind, naked, and feeling no pain. *The Anatomical Record.* 303:77–88.

Burrell BD. (2017) Comparative biology of pain: What invertebrates can tell us about how nociception works. *J Neurophysiol.* Apr 1; 117(4):1461-1473.

Bushnell MC, Ceko M, Low LA. (2013) Cognitive and emotional control of pain and its disruption in chronic pain. *Nat Rev Neurosci.* Jul; 14(7):502-11.

Butler D, Moseley L. (2020) *Explain Pain* (Second edition). Noigroup Publications.

Cela-Conde CJ, Lombardo RG, Avise JC, Ayala FJ. (2014) *In the Light of Evolution: Volume VII: The Human Mental Machinery.* Washington (DC): National Academies Press (US).

Chaudhury R et al. (2024) Mycorrhization in trees: Ecology, physiology, emerging technologies and beyond. *Plant Biol* (Stuttg). Mar; 26(2):145-156.

Cohen M, Quintner J, Buchanan D. (2013) Is chronic pain a disease? *Pain Med.* Sep; 14(9):1284-8.

Corballis MC. (2009) The evolution of language. *Ann N Y Acad Sci.* Mar; 1156:19-43.

Damasio A. (2019) De vergissing van Descartes: Gevoel, verstand en het menselijk brein [Eng: Descartes error] (Dutch Edition). Wereldbibliotheek.

Damasio AR. (2000) *The Feeling of What Happens.* Vintage.

Darwin CR. (1859) *On the Origin of Species by Means of Natural Selection, or the Preservation of Favoured Races in the Struggle for Life.* London: John Murray.

Monkey Business

Darwin CR. (1872) *The Expression of the Emotions in Man and Animals*. London: John Murray.

Davies NB, Krebs JR, West SA. (2012) *An Introduction to Behavioural Ecology*. Wiley.

De la Fuente MF, Souto A, Albuquerque UP, Schiel N. (2022) Self-medication in nonhuman primates: A systematic evaluation of the possible function of the use of medicinal plants. *Am J Primatol*. Nov; 84(11):e23438.

de Waal F. (2019) Zijn we slim genoeg om te weten hoe slim dieren zijn? [Eng: Are We Smart Enough to Know How Smart Animals Are?] (13de editie). Olympus.

de Waal FBM, Berger ML. (2000) Payment for labour in monkeys. *Nature*. Vol. 4.

de Waal FB, Suchak M. (2010) Prosocial primates: Selfish and unselfish motivations. *Philos Trans R Soc Lond B Biol Sci*. Sep 12; 365(1553):2711-22.

de Waal FB. (2008) Putting the altruism back into altruism: The evolution of empathy. *Annu Rev Psychol*. 59:279-300.

de Waal FBM, Preston SD. (2017) Mammalian empathy: Behavioural manifestations and neural basis. *Nat Rev Neurosci*. Aug; 18(8):498-509.

Driessen HGGM. (2002) Pijn en cultuur [Eng: pain and culture]/ druk 2. Wereldbibliotheek.

Edwards RR, Dworkin RH, Sullivan MD, Turk DC, Wasan AD. (2016) The role of psychosocial processes in the development and maintenance of chronic pain. *J Pain.* Sep; 17(9) Suppl:T70-92.

Elma M, Yilmaz ST, Deliens T, Coppieters I, Clarys P, Nijs J, Malfliet A. (2020) Do nutritional factors interact with chronic musculoskeletal pain? A systematic review. *J Clin Med.* 9(3):702.

Engel GL. (2012) The need for a new medical model: A challenge for biomedicine. *Psychodyn Psychiatry.* Sep; 40(3):377-96.

Ferguson G. (2019) De acht grote lessen van de natuur [Eng : Eight Master Lessons of Nature](1ste editie). Ten Have.

Flor H, Diers M. (2009) Sensorimotor training and cortical reorganization. *NeuroRehabilitation.* 25(1):19-27.

Flor H. (2012) New developments in the understanding and management of persistent pain. *Curr Opin Psychiatry.* 25:109–113.

Flor H. (2003) Remapping somatosensory cortex after injury. *Adv Neurol.* 93:195-204.

Fowler A, Koutsioni Y, Sommer V. (2007) Leaf-swallowing in Nigerian chimpanzees: Evidence for assumed self-medication. *Primates.* Jan; 48(1):73-6.

Frank ET, Buffat D, Liberti J, Aibekova L, Economo EP, Keller L. (2024) Wound-dependent leg amputations to combat infections in an ant society. *Curr Biol.* Jul 22; 34(14):3273-3278.e3.

Frijda N. (1988) *The Emotions.* Cambridge University Press.

Galef BG. (2013) Imitation and local enhancement: Detrimental effects of consensus definitions on analyses of social learning in animals. *Behav Processes.* Nov; 100:123-30.

Garcia-Larrea L et al. (2018) Pain and consciousness: *Progress in neuro-psycho pharmacology & biological psychiatry.* 87:193-199.
Ghaemi N. (2010) *The Rise and Fall of the Biopsychosocial Model. Reconciling Art and Science in Psychiatry.* Johns Hopkins University Press.

Gilam G, Gross JJ, Wager TD, Keefe FJ, Mackey SC. (2020) What is the relationship between pain and emotion? Bridging constructs and communities. *Neuron.* Jul 8; 107(1):17-21.

Godfrey-Smith P. (2016) Buitengewoon bewustzijn: de octopus en de evolutie van de intelligentie. [Other

Minds The Octopus and the Evolution of Intelligent Life] Unieboek | Het Spectrum.

Goldberg DS, McGee SJ. (2011) Pain as a global public health priority. *BMC Public Health.* Oct 6; 11:770.

Gray H, Carter HV. (2007) *Gray's Anatomy: A Facsimile* (Facsimile edition). New Line Books.

Graziano MSA, Webb TW. (2017) From Sponge to Human: The Evolution of Consciousness. In: Kaas, J (ed.), *Evolution of Nervous Systems* 2e. Vol. 3, pp. 547–554. Oxford: Elsevier.

Greene AM, Panyadee P, Inta A, Huffman MA. (2020) Asian elephant self-medication as a source of ethnoveterinary knowledge among Karen mahouts in northern Thailand. *J Ethnopharmacol.* Sep 15; 259:112823.

Gustin Syliva M et al. (2012) Pain and plasticity: Is chronic pain always associated with somatosensory cortex activity and reorganization? *J Neurosci.* Oct 24; 32(43):14874–14884.

Gutfreund Y. (2018) The mind-evolution problem: The difficulty of fitting consciousness in an evolutionary framework. *Front Psychol.* Aug 24; 9:1537.

Hanyu-Deutmeyer AA, Cascella M, Varacallo M. (2023) *Phantom Limb Pain.* StatPearls, Treasure Island (FL): StatPearls Publishing.

Harari YN. (2015) *Sapiens.* HarperCollins.

Hassan S, Muere A, Einstein G. (2014) Ovarian hormones and chronic pain: A comprehensive review. *Pain.* 155(12), 2448–2460.

Hawkins RD, Greene W, Kandel ER. (1998) Classical conditioning, differential conditioning, and second-order conditioning of the Aplysia gill-withdrawal reflex in a simplified mantle organ preparation. *Behav Neurosci.* Jun; 112(3):636-45.

He J, Li B, Han S, Zhang Y, Liu K, Yi S, Liu Y, Xiu M. (2022) Drosophila as a model to study the mechanism of nociception. *Front Physiol.* Mar 28; 13:854124.

Heyes C. (2012) New thinking: The evolution of human cognition. *Philos Trans R Soc Lond B Biol Sci.* Aug 5; 367(1599):2091-6.

Heyes CM. (1994) Social learning in animals: Categories and mechanisms. *Biol Rev Camb Philos Soc.* May; 69(2):207-31.

Huffman M. (1997) Current evidence for self-medication in primates: A multidisciplinary perspective. *Yearb Phys Anthropol.* 104:171–200.

Huffman MA, Page JE, Sukhdeo MVK et al. (1996) Leaf-swallowing by chimpanzees: A behavioural adaptation for the control of strongyle nematode infections. *Int J Primatol.* 17:475–503.

Im SH, Galko MJ. (2012) Pokes, sunburn, and hot sauce: Drosophila as an emerging model for the biology of nociception. *Dev Dyn.* Jan; 241(1):16-26.
Loeser JD, Melzack R. (1999) Pain: An overview. *Lancet.* 353:1607–09.

Kabat-Zinn J. (2013) *Full Catastrophe Living.* Piatkus Books.

Kandel ER. (2000) The molecular biology of memory storage: A dialog between genes and synapses. *Nobel Lecture.* December 8.

Kaufman AB, Call J, Kaufman, JC. (2021) *The Cambridge Handbook of Animal Cognition* (Cambridge Handbooks in Psychology). Cambridge University Press.

Kaur A, Guan Y. (2018) Phantom limb pain: A literature review. *Chin J Traumatol.* Dec; 21(6):366-368.

Keefe FJ, Lumley MA, Buffington AL, Carson JW, Studts JL, Edwards CL, Macklem DJ, Aspnes AK, Fox L, Steffey D. (2002) Changing face of pain: Evolution of pain research in psychosomatic medicine. *Psychosom Med.* Nov-Dec; 64(6):921-38.

Klein S. (2014) *Survival of the Nicest: How Altruism Made Us Human and Why It Pays to Get Along.* Scribe UK.

Koke A et al. (2022) Chronische pijn en het bio psychosociale model. [Eng: Chronic pain and the biopsychosocial model] Nervus. Dec; Nummer 4.

Kuner R, Flor H. (2016) Structural plasticity and reorganisation in chronic pain. *Nat Rev Neurosci.* Dec 15; 18(1):20-30.

Levy RL, Langer SL, Whitehead WE. (2007) Social learning contributions to the etiology and treatment of functional abdominal pain and inflammatory bowel disease in children and adults. *World J Gastroenterol.* May 7; (17):2397-403.

Makin TR, Flor H. (2020) Brain (re)organisation following amputation: Implications for phantom limb pain. *Neuroimage.* Sep; 218:116943.

Mascaro A, Southern LM, Deschner T, Pika S. (2022) Application of insects to wounds of self and others by chimpanzees in the wild. *Curr Biol.* Feb 7; 32(3):R112-R113.

Masi S, Gustafsson E, Saint Jalme M, Narat V, Todd A, Bomsel MC, Krief S. (2012) Unusual feeding behaviour in wild great apes, a window to understand origins of self-medication in humans:

Role of sociality and physiology on learning process. *Physiol Behav.* Jan 18; 105(2):337-49.

McLennan MR, Hasegawa H, Bardi M, Huffman MA. (2017) Gastrointestinal parasite infections and self-medication in wild chimpanzees surviving in degraded forest fragments within an agricultural landscape mosaic in Uganda. *PLoS One.* Jul 10; 12(7):e0180431.

Mease P. (2005) Fibromyalgia syndrome: Review of clinical presentation, pathogenesis, outcome measures, and treatment. *J Rheumatol Suppl.* Aug; 75:6-21.

Melzack R, Wall PD. (1965) Pain mechanisms: A new theory. *Science.* Nov 19; 150(3699):971-9.

Moayedi M, Davis KD. (2013) Theories of pain: From specificity to gate control. *J Neurophysiol.* Jan; 109(1):5-12.

Mogil JS. (2019) The translatability of pain across species. *Phil. Trans. R. Soc. B.* 374:20190286.

Morree JJ. (2008) Dynamiek van het menselijk bindweefsel. [Dynamics of human connective tissue] Bohn Stafleu van Loghum.

Moseley G, Butler DS. (2015) Fifteen years of explaining pain: The past, present, and future. *J Pain.* 16(9):807–813.

Moseley GL. (2004) Does anticipation of back pain predispose to back trouble? *Brain.* 127(10):2339–2347.

Nesse RM, Schulkin J. (2019) An evolutionary medicine perspective on pain and its disorders. *Phil. Trans. R. Soc. B.* 374

Nesse RM, Schulkin J. (2019) An evolutionary medicine perspective on pain and its disorders. *Philos Trans R Soc Lond B Biol Sci.* Nov 11; 374(1785).

Nijs J et al (2011) How to explain central sensitization to patients with 'unexplained' chronic musculoskeletal pain: Practice guidelines. *Manual Therapy.* 16:413e418.

Obbo CJ, Makanga B, Mulholland DA, Coombes PH, Brun R. (2013) Antiprotozoal activity of Khaya anthotheca, (Welv.) C.D.C. a plant used by chimpanzees for self-medication. *J Ethnopharmacol.* May 2; 147(1):220-3.

Pattison LA, Callejo G, St John Smith E. (2019) Evolution of acid nociception: Ion channels and receptors for detecting acid. *Philos Trans R Soc Lond B Biol Sci.* Nov 11; 374(1785).

Peters ML. (2015) Emotional and cognitive influences on pain experience. *Mod Trends Pharmacopsychiatry.* 30:138-52.

Petkov CI, Ten Cate C. (2020) Structured sequence learning: Animal abilities, cognitive operations, and language evolution. *Top Cogn Sci.* Jul; 12(3):828-842.

Raffaeli W, Tenti M, Corraro A, Malafoglia V, Ilari S, Balzani E, Bonci A. (2021) Chronic pain: What does it mean? A review on the use of the term chronic pain in clinical practice. *J Pain Res.* Mar 29; 14:827-835.

Reesink M. (2021) Dier en mens: De band tussen ons en andere dieren. [Animal and human. The bond between us and other animals] Boom.

Schleip R, Stecco C, Driscoll M, Huijing P. (2012) *Fascia: The Tensional Network of the Human Body: The science and clinical applications in manual and movement therapy* (1st edition). Churchill Livingstone.

Schone HR, Baker CI, Katz J, Nikolajsen L, Limakatso K, Flor H, Makin TR. (2022) Making sense of phantom limb pain. *J Neurol Neurosurg Psychiatry.* May 24; 93(8):833–43.

Seksel K. (2007) *How Pain Affects Animals.* Australian Animal Welfare Strategy Science Summit on Pain and Pain Management, Proceedings.

Sirianni J, Ibrahim M, Patwardhan A. (2015) Chronic pain syndromes, mechanisms, and current treatments. *Prog Mol Biol Transl Sci.* 131:565-611.

Smith ES, Lewin GR. (2009) Nociceptors: a phylogenetic view. *J Comp Physiol A Neuroethol Sens Neural Behav Physiol.* Dec; 195(12):1089-106.

Smith ESJ, Park TJ, Lewin GR. (2020) Independent evolution of pain insensitivity in African mole-rats: Origins and mechanisms. *J Comp Physiol A Neuroethol Sens Neural Behav Physiol.* May; 206(3):313-325.

Sneddon LU, Braithwaite VA, Gentle MJ. (2003) Do fish have nociceptors? Evidence for the evolution of a vertebrate sensory system. *Proc Biol Sci.* Jun 7; 270(1520):1115-21.

Sneddon LU. (2004) Evolution of nociception in vertebrates: Comparative analysis of lower vertebrates. *Brain Res Brain Res Rev.* Oct; 46(2):123-30.

Sneddon LU. (2019) Evolution of nociception and pain: Evidence from fish models. *Philos Trans R Soc Lond B Biol Sci.* Nov 11; 374(1785):20190290.

Sneddon LU. (2018) Comparative physiology of nociception and pain. *Physiology* (Bethesda). Jan 1; 33(1):63-73.

Swaab DF. (2011) Wij zijn ons brein [Eng: We are our brain] (Amsterdam/Antwerpen, Uitgeverij Contact, 2008–2011, ed. Contact)

Turner SE et al. (2014) Social consequences of disability in a nonhuman primate. *J Hum Evol.* 68:47-57.

Van Cranenburgh, B. (2009) Toegepaste neurowetenschappen 3 - Pijn. [Eng: Applied neurosciences] Reed Business Education.

Van Dieën JH, Hodges PW, Cholewicki J. (2013) *Spinal Control.* Elsevier Gezondheidszorg.

Van Wingerden JP. (2014) Rugpijn En Andere Onbegrepen Klachten. [Eng: Backpain and other poorly understood complaints] Bohn Stafleu van Loghum.

Vlaeyen JWS, Crombez G, Linton SJ. (2016) The fear-avoidance model of pain. *Pain.* Aug; 157(8):1588-1589.

Vlaeyen JWS, Kole-Snijders AMJ, Boeren RGB, van Eek H. (1995) Fear of movement/(re)injury in chronic low back pain and its relation to behavioural performance. *Pain.* Sep; 62(3):363-372.

Vleeming A, Mooney V, Stoeckart R. (2007) *Movement, Stability & Lumbopelvic Pain: Integration of research and therapy* (2nd edition). Churchill Livingstone.

Waddel G. (2004) *The Back Pain Revolution* (2nd edition). Churchill Livingstone.

Wall, P. (2001) Pijn (1ste editie) [Eng: Pain]. SWP.

Walters ET, Carew TJ, Kandel ER. (1979) Classical conditioning in Aplysia californica. *Proc Natl Acad Sci USA*. Dec; 76(12):6675-9.

Walters ET, Williams ACC. (2019) Evolution of mechanisms and behaviour important for pain. *Philos Trans R Soc Lond B Biol Sci*. Nov 11; 374(1785):20190275.

Walters ET. (2019) Adaptive mechanisms driving maladaptive pain: How chronic ongoing activity in primary nociceptors can enhance evolutionary fitness after severe injury. *Phil. Trans. R. Soc. B.* 374.

Wang X, Tedford R, Antón M. (2010) *Dogs: Their Fossil Relatives and Evolutionary History* (Illustrated edition). Columbia University Press.

Whitehead H, Rendell L. (2015) *The Cultural Lives of Whales and Dolphins*. University of Chicago Press.

Wich SA, Atmoko SUS, Setia TM, Schaik CVP. (2010) *Orangutans: Geographic Variation in Behavioural Ecology and Conservation* (Illustrated edition). Oxford University Press.

Williams AC. (2019) Persistence of pain in humans and other mammals. *Phil. Trans. R. Soc. B.* 374:20190276.

Wohlleben P. (2016) *The Hidden Life of Trees, What They Feel, How They Communicate.* Greystone books. Vancouver/Berkeley.

Woolf CJ. (2010) What is this thing called pain? *J Clin Invest.* Nov; 120(11):3742-4.

Yu JG, Carlsson L, Thornell LE. (2004) Evidence for myofibril remodeling as opposed to myofibril damage in human muscles with DOMS: An ultrastructural and immunoelectron microscopic study. *Histochem Cell Biol.* Mar; 121(3):219-27.

Zentall TR. (2006) Imitation: Definitions, evidence, and mechanisms. *Anim Cogn.* Oct; 9(4):335-53.

Zimmer Z, Fraser K, Grol-Prokopczyk H, Zajacova A. (2022) A global study of pain prevalence across 52 countries: Examining the role of country-level contextual factors. *Pain.* Sep 1; 163(9):1740-1750.

Zorgstandaard Chronische Pijn [Eng: Standard of care for chronic pain], 28 Maart 2017.

Monkey Business

Acknowledgements

Vince: 'Shouldn't we include a word of thanks?'

JP: 'We tried, but it turned into a melancholic drama.'

Vince: 'Yes, that was a bit too much of a good thing. But we owe a lot to other people, don't we? We can't leave that unmentioned.'

JP: 'You've got a point there. For example, I'm thinking of all the people with pain complaints that we've seen over the years. And the discussions and conversations with our fellow practitioners.'

Vince: 'And don't forget all the animals that I've been able to treat in recent years...'

JP: 'Yes, yes, they're part of it, too. Although they probably don't care much.'

Vince: 'Yes, that's what you think... And is it going too far to mention those high-level scientists?'

JP: 'Well, Darwin has been gone for a long time, just like Nico Frijda, and our hero in this field, Frans de Waal, also passed away recently. I learned a lot from his insights in his books.'

Vince: 'I also think of Niko Tinbergen, Jane Goodall, Louis Leaky, Melzack & Wall and Yuval Noah Harari. I learned a lot from them, too. And do we still have family and friends?'

JP: 'Family is family. They are an essential part of it and without family, we and the book would not exist. But there are still a number of people who really contributed to the book: Andrea, Hans and Samragi, who struggled through the first English version; Kirsten, our English editor; Richard our thorough proofreader; Wilma, who removed our language errors from the Dutch version. And Gert-Jan, who always gives us wise advice.'

Vince: 'And don't forget Bernadette, who provided the beautiful illustration for the cover.'

Vince & JP: 'To everyone who contributed in one way or another: many thanks, even if we chaotic people accidentally forgot to mention you.'

Vince: 'Oh since I love to have the last word, you know me... Special thanks to Jeffrey, for his love and all and because I forgot to mention him in the first Dutch edition...'

www.ingramcontent.com/pod-product-compliance
Lightning Source LLC
LaVergne TN
LVHW041645070526
838199LV00053B/3566